# The Trophoblast and the Origins of Cancer

# The Trophoblast and the Origins of Cancer

*One solution to the
medical enigma of our time*

**Nicholas J. Gonzalez, M.D.**
**Linda L. Isaacs, M.D.**

NEW SPRING PRESS

# Notice

This book is intended for general informational purposes only, not as a medical manual. The materials presented in no way are meant to be a substitute for professional medical care or attention by a qualified practitioner, nor should they be construed as such. Always check with your doctor if you have any questions or concerns about your condition or before starting or modifying a program of treatment. New Spring Press LLC and the author(s) are not responsible or liable, directly or indirectly, for any form of damages whatsoever resulting from the use (or misuse) of information contained in or implied by this book.

Book design by Anne M. Landgraf, Brooklyn BookWorks LLC.

Publisher's Cataloging-in-Publication
*(Provided by Quality Books, Inc.)*

Gonzalez, Nicholas J.
   The trophoblast and the origins of cancer : one solution to the medical enigma of our time / Nicholas J. Gonzalez and Linda L. Isaacs.
      p. cm.
   Includes bibliographical references and index.
   LCCN 2009935675
   ISBN-13: 978-0-9821965-0-2
   ISBN-10: 0-9821965-0-4
   1. Cancer—Etiology.   2. Cancer—Treatment.   3. Trophoblast.   I. Isaacs, Linda L.
II. Title.
   RC268.48.G66 2009                                          616.99'4071
                                                              QBI09-600149

Text excerpts reprinted from *Seminars in Reproductive Endocrinology,* Volume 17, Murray MJ, Lessey BA, Embryo implantation and tumor metastasis: common pathways of invasion and angiogenesis, Pages 275–290, Copyright 1999, with permission from Thieme Medical Publishers.

Text excerpts reprinted from *Cancer: Principles & Practice of Oncology,* 6th Edition, DeVita VT, Jr., Hellman S, Rosenberg SA, editors, Stetler-Stevenson WG, Kleiner DE, Molecular biology of cancer: invasion and metastases, Pages 127–134, Copyright 2001, with permission from Lippincott Williams & Wilkins.

Text excerpt reprinted from *Stem Cells,* Volume 21, Turnpenny L, Brickwood S, Spalluto CM et al. Derivation of human embryonic germ cells: an alternative source of pluripotent stem cells, Pages 598–609, Copyright 2003, with permission from AlphaMed Press.

Text excerpt reprinted from *U-M Comprehensive Cancer Center News,* Pobojewski S, U-M scientists find "stem cells" in human breast cancer, http://www.cancer.med.umich.edu/news/stemcell.htm, Copyright 2003, with permission from the University of Michigan Comprehensive Cancer Center.

Text excerpts reprinted from *Oncology News International,* Volume 15, Growing evidence supports stem cell hypothesis of cancer, Pages 24–25, Copyright 2006, with permission from Oncology News International.

Text excerpts reprinted from *Gastroenterology,* Volume 108, Terada T, Nakanuma Y, Expression of pancreatic enzymes (α-amylase, trypsinogen, and lipase) during human liver development and maturation, Pages 1236–1245, Copyright 1995, with permission from Elsevier.

Text excerpts reprinted from *Physiological Reviews,* Volume 82, Rothman S, Liebow C, Isenman L, Conservation of digestive enzymes, Pages 1–18, Copyright 2002 American Physiological Society, permission conveyed through Copyright Clearance Center, Inc.

**To the memory of Dr. John Beard (1858–1924)**

He fought the good fight in defense of scientific truth,

and for the benefit of cancer patients everywhere.

# Contents

# Acknowledgements

Many people have contributed in many ways over the years, to help support and develop our treatment, and specifically to help this book see the light of day. As a start I would like to thank my current devoted staff, Chelsea Leinberger and Angela Rios, who have reviewed this book carefully through its various drafts, offering many useful and thoughtful suggestions.

I would like to extend an extra special thanks to my friend and supporter Pierre Guesry, M.D., the now retired former Vice President for Research at Nestle, who long ago believed in the value of our treatment and persuaded Nestle to fund our first clinical and animal studies. I would like to thank J.P. Jones, Ph.D., the retired former Vice President for Research in Health Care at The Procter & Gamble Company. JP approved the funding that allowed us to finalize the manufacturing process for our particular enzymes, a major undertaking, and a major contribution to our therapy. Even in retirement, he remains a good friend and much valued advisor to our research efforts.

I wish to thank Suzanne Somers, who has done so much over the years to get the word out about alternative medicine, and whose new book *Knockout* features our treatment approach along with a number of our patients diagnosed with poor prognosis or terminal cancer.

My friend Hans Moolenburg, M.D., in my opinion one of the finest physicians in Europe or anywhere else, has been a strong supporter and guide through both difficult and good times over the years, and remains the finest Bible scholar I've ever met.

I owe much to Jonathan Wright, M.D., whose columns in the old *Prevention Magazine* I used to read with anticipation, in those days before I had even gone to medical school. He too, has helped me over the years, in a number of ways. I appreciate enormously the work of Sally Fallon Morell, who has done so much to promote the concepts of good fats, healthy soil, and organic small farming, and who has worked ceaselessly to keep the work and writings of Weston Price, D.D.S. alive and vital. I am grateful for the opportunity to speak at her national conferences, this year to be held (fall 2009) in Illinois. I have multiple copies of her cookbook, *Nourishing Traditions*, which I refer to regularly and recommend to anybody and everybody with an interest in nutrition.

Sir Roger Norrington, the internationally acclaimed English orchestral conductor and my friend, has not only been an inspiration, in overcoming the obstacles he has faced in his own professional life—bias against truth isn't limited to the scientific realm—but has offered great wisdom, in terms of overcoming the indifference and scorn of recalcitrant colleagues.

Judith Pryor, with great editorial insight, worked long and hard on various drafts, offering many useful suggestions on style and organization.

And of course, I wish to thank my wife Mary Beth, who has lived through years of my hard work with virtually no complaining, enduring my writing late into the night and on weekends and putting vacations aside as I toiled on my various writing projects, the first of which is this book. It isn't always fun, being married to a driven, hardworking physician-scientist who seems to have been placed in the position of taking on the academic medical universe, but she understands completely the seriousness, and ultimate value, of this difficult and consuming task.

Nicholas J. Gonzalez, M.D.

# PART I

# The Trophoblast as Metaphor for Cancer

# Introduction to Part I

Over the past ten years, a number of cancer researchers have turned their attention to the non-malignant trophoblast, the embryonic tissue that develops into the mammalian placenta, the connection between the growing fetus in pregnancy and the maternal uterus.[1;2] Certainly, in its earliest incarnation as a relatively undifferentiated cell line capable of rapid proliferation, invasion into nearby tissues, migration, and new blood vessel formation, the trophoblast does resemble a typical aggressive neoplasm in its general behavior, and would seem to serve as an ideal model for the study of malignancy. Indeed, the similarities between cancer and trophoblast, as we continue to learn, go deep, right to the level of molecular mechanisms that define each of these two cell types, the one completely normal and necessary for human life, the other dreaded and deadly in its potential.

A recent article entitled "Molecular circuits shared by placental and cancer cells, and their implications in the proliferative, invasive and migratory capacities of trophoblasts" catalogues in elegant detail the biochemical pathways, the signaling and enzymatic processes shared by both trophoblasts and malignancy.[2] In the introduction of this 2007 publication, the authors summarize their thesis of a fundamental identity between the trophoblast and cancer:

> Although the placenta is a normal tissue, its constituent cells, the trophoblastic cells, share several common features with

malignant cells. Their high cell proliferation, their lack of cell-contact inhibition, their migratory and invasive properties as well as their capacity to escape effectors of the immune system, in particular during the first trimester of pregnancy, have led to the definition of the trophoblast as a "pseudo-malignant" type of tissue or as a "physiological metastasis" . . . [2]

One hundred years earlier, long before the current resurgence of interest in the subject, in a series of long forgotten articles and in his 1911 book, *The Enzyme Treatment of Cancer*, the biologist Dr. John Beard working at the University of Edinburgh first proposed the trophoblast as the ideal model of cancer.[3] In his writings, Dr. Beard actually went quite a bit further than mere similarity between the two tissue lines, suggesting that the trophoblast not only resembled malignant tissue in its appearance and activity, but was the very cell line from which all cancer developed—and the only cell from which malignancy could form.

Beard claimed, as part of his trophoblast as cancer hypothesis, that nests of germ cells, the precursors in adults to gametes, remained scattered throughout all of our tissues, the remnants of their peculiar migration from the yolk sac to the developing gonads in the early embryo. Normally, such germ cells remain quiescent, but if stimulated into activity, they can develop as aberrant gametes, complete with their own trophoblast. Dr. Beard believed this "vagrant" trophoblast, growing out of place can, if unchecked, form malignancy.

Beard's colleagues during his lifetime had little tolerance for his startling hypotheses, which they rejected out of hand as simply preposterous. When Beard died in 1924, he died in obscurity, his ideas about the trophoblast as the model for and actual origin of cancer long forgotten. But with the current growing interest among academicians who see in the trophoblast the ideal cancer analogy, we can think of no better time than the 150th anniversary of Dr. Beard's birth to reassess his thesis from the perspective of contemporary molecular biology.

# CHAPTER 1

# Trophoblast Implantation—
# an Overview

As we venture into Dr. Beard's trophoblastic hypothesis, we will begin with a review of modern concepts about implantation of the early embryo into the uterine lining. For much of the next section we have relied on two excellent sources. The first, *Human Embryology and Developmental Biology*, by Bruce Carlson, M.D., Ph.D., of the University of Michigan,[4] brings embryology away from the purely descriptive and into the modern world of molecular biology. The second reference, a summary of contemporary thinking about embryonic implantation and placental growth, appeared in the *New England Journal of Medicine* on November 8, 2001.[5]

Conception and implantation of the embryo with its trophoblast into the uterine lining involves a precise orchestration of various endocrine glands, the hormones they produce, and the organs they influence, including the uterus and the embryo itself, all within a short period of several days.[5-7] The whole process really begins in the ovaries lying on either side of the pelvis, which perform two major functions critical for new life: first, they provide the eggs, which if fertilized become the embryo. Second, the active ovarian follicles secrete estrogen and progesterone, the two hormones responsible for helping regulate the ovulatory cycle.[4]

Each ovary lies adjacent to a fimbria, the fan-like tip of the Fallopian tube which serves as a conduit to carry eggs from the ovaries to the uterine cavity itself. The fimbria do not come into direct contact with the

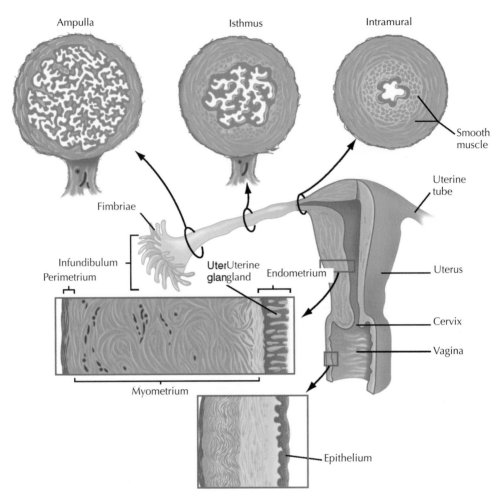

**FIGURE 1:** Structure of the female reproductive tract.

*(Originally published in Carlson BM: Human Embryology & Developmental Biology, 4th Ed., St. Louis, Mosby, 2008. Copyright Mosby 2008. Used with permission.)*

ovaries but lie a short distance from them so that after its release, the egg must travel this distance before entering one of the two tubes.

The uterus, shaped like an inverted pear sitting in the middle of the pelvis, consists of a central cavity lined by the endometrium, normally some 5–6 mm wide, with a thick muscle layer beneath, the muscularis (See Figure 1).[4(p15)] A layer of columnar epithelial cells lines the surface of the endometrium directly facing the uterine cavity, attached at their base to a basement membrane, a type of biological cement consisting of collagen and glycoproteins. This structure serves as a foundation for the epithelium, as well as a barrier between it and the underlying tissues.

A layer of thick connective tissue, the stroma, consisting of coiled proteins and collagen, lies directly beneath the columnar layer and its associated basement membrane,[4(p15-16)] and beneath this lie the thick muscular layers of the myometrium. The stroma contains a variety of structures such as the spiral arteries and veins as well as the uterine glands, microscopic sacs lined by an epithelium responsible for secreting mucus and nutritive substances to support an implanted embryo. The spiral vessels, specialized outgrowths from the main uterine arteries and veins, not only provide the circulation to feed the endometrial tissues, but serve, should implantation succeed, as the point of contact between the blood supply of the mother and that of the growing embryo.

During the tissue shedding of menstruation, the spiral arteries constrict, reducing blood supply to the uterine surface so that in turn, most of the endometrial lining, with the exception of a thick basilar layer of cells, dies and sloughs off. Immediately after menstruation, under the influence of estrogen secreted into the bloodstream by the ovary, the remaining cells within this basal tissue begin dividing rapidly, forming a replacement endometrium with its distinctive cell layers.[4(pp16-20)]

Menstrual shedding occurs if the egg from the previous cycle remains unfertilized, or if fertilized, fails to implant into the uterine lining and dies. In this circumstance, the ovarian follicle atrophies, so that estrogen and progesterone levels fall precipitously. In response to low circulating estrogen, the anterior portion of the pituitary, a small gland located at the base of the brain, releases follicular stimulating hormone (FSH). This protein acts directly on the ovaries to stimulate a number of dormant eggs, estimated in the range of 20–50, to begin maturing. As pituitary FSH secretion rises, the active ovarian follicles increase their synthesis of estrogen and its release into the systemic circulation. Estrogen in turn stimulates the rapid regrowth of the denuded endometrial lining, preparing it once again to accept a fertilized egg.[4(pp16-20)]

During the first two weeks of the cycle, technically known as the proliferative phase to reflect the regeneration processes at work, all but one of the 20-50 activated ovarian follicles gradually atrophy, reducing to little more than minute areas of scar tissue. The remaining active follicle, with the vital egg in its core, continues secreting estrogen, the levels of which stay moderately high and then rapidly peak 24 hours before day 14, the midpoint of the cycle. This estrogen flood signals steroid-sensitive cells in the hypothalamus, a portion of the lower brain connected to the pituitary gland (See Figure 2). These cells in turn direct the anterior pituitary to release large amounts of both FSH and a second protein, luteinizing hormone (LH). For 24 hours on and around day 14, levels of these two hormones reach their highest levels of the entire 28 day cycle, with FSH increasing about two fold, and LH rising more significantly, about eight fold. [4(pp16-20)]

As a result of the LH surge on day 14, the follicle—now called the corpus luteum—dramatically changes character, releasing less estrogen but considerably more progesterone, needed to prepare the uterine lining so that it can effectively accept a viable embryo. During the latter two weeks of the cycle, termed the secretory phase, under the influence of progesterone the endometrial glands begin synthesizing considerable amounts of glycogen and other nutritive substances to provide sustenance for an implanted fertilized egg. At the same time, the spiral arteries begin growing rapidly throughout the endometrium, providing the blood supply needed should an embryo attach.

In response to rising LH blood levels, the one remaining viable egg emerges from the ovary, then makes its way to the adjacent Fallopian tube. At this point, the newly released egg consists of a single central cell protected by an outer coating of cells, the corona radiata, and an inner, microscopically thin protein shell, the zona pellucida (See Figure 3). Once in the tube the corona radiata quickly deteriorates, leaving only the pellucida layer. At this point, the egg, if not fertilized within the next 12–24 hours, will shrivel up and die.[4(pp24-26)]

Meanwhile, progesterone, now abundant, readies the Fallopian tube to receive and transport the newly released egg. Under its influence, beginning on day 14 of the cycle the tube contracts rhythmically, while its ep-

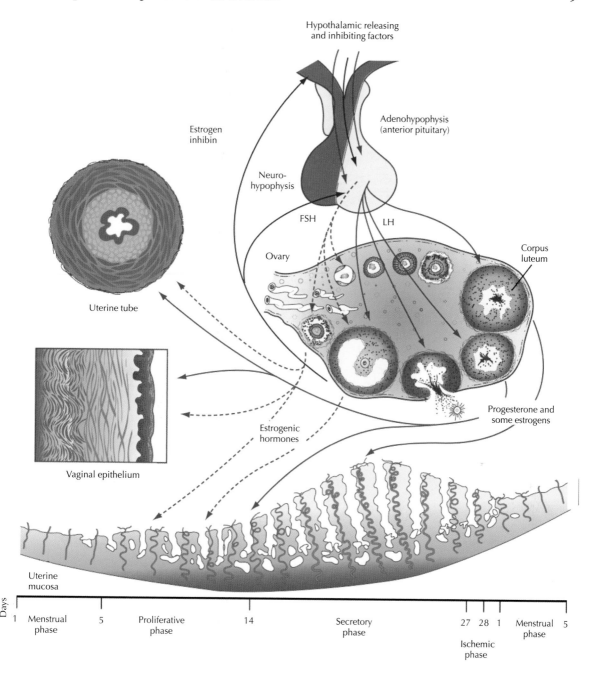

Hypothalamic releasing
and inhibiting factors

Adenohypophysis
(anterior pituitary)

Estrogen
inhibin

Neuro-
hypophysis

FSH

LH

Corpus
luteum

Ovary

Uterine tube

Progesterone and
some estrogens

Estrogenic
hormones

Vaginal epithelium

Uterine
mucosa

Days

| 1 | Menstrual phase | 5 | Proliferative phase | 14 | Secretory phase | 27 28 1 | Menstrual phase | 5 |

Ischemic
phase

**FIGURE 2:** General scheme of hormonal control of reproduction in the female.

*(Originally published in Carlson BM: Human Embryology & Developmental Biology, 4th Ed., St. Louis, Mosby, 2008. Copyright Mosby 2008. Used with permission.)*

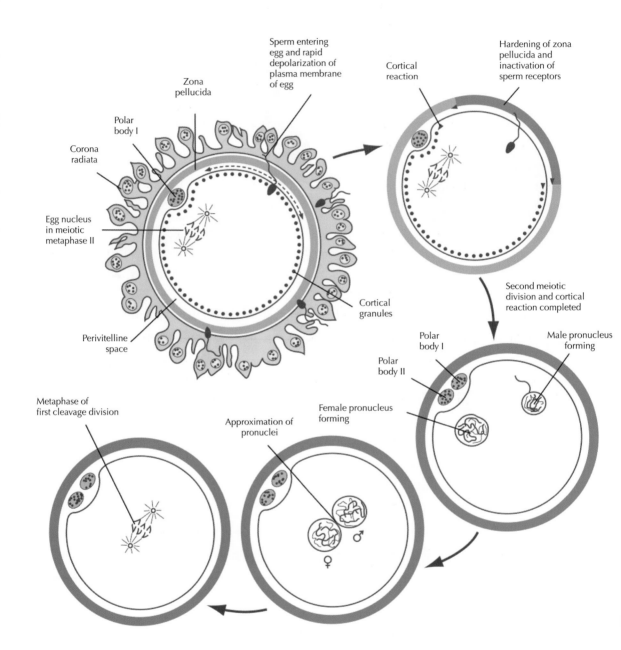

**FIGURE 3:** Summary of the main events involved in fertilization.

*(Originally published in Carlson BM: Human Embryology & Developmental Biology, 4<sup>th</sup> Ed., St. Louis, Mosby, 2008. Copyright Mosby 2008. Used with permission.)*

ithelium secretes a nutritionally rich fluid to nourish the egg as it moves toward the uterus.[4(pp16-20)]

Overall, the journey of an egg through the Fallopian tube into the uterine cavity takes a total of about three days. As the egg reaches the uterus, the high levels of circulating progesterone feed back to the hypothalamus, which then signals the anterior pituitary to reduce secretion of LH (See Figure 4). If fertilization and implantation fail, the corpus luteum (the remaining active ovarian follicle) secretes inhibin, a hormone that further blocks LH release.[4(p19)] In turn, progesterone levels drop rapidly so that during the last three or four days of the cycle, the blood concentrations of the two pituitary hormones, FSH and LH, along with the two ovarian hormones, estrogen and progesterone, fall to their lowest point of the cycle. In response to the decline in circulating progesterone, the spiral arteries involute, reducing blood flow to the endometrium. With the supply of nutrients and oxygen cut off, the endometrial cells undergo apoptosis (programmed cell death) before sloughing off during the first days of menstruation. At the beginning of the new cycle, the hypothalamus responds to the low estrogen levels by signaling the anterior pituitary to resume its synthesis and release of FSH, which stimulates the next generation of ovarian follicles into action. In turn, estrogen levels start to climb as the cycle starts anew.

If fertilized, the egg begins dividing even while traversing the Fallopian tube, increasing first to two cells then to three, then to four, each cell totipotential, that is, able to form an entire embryo (See Figure 5). By the time the proliferating egg reaches the uterine cavity it consists of a tiny ball of 12–16 cells, referred to as the morula, the Latin name for mulberry in deference to its resemblance to that particular fruit.[5] The cells of the morula appear identical, primitive, and undifferentiated but have lost their totipotentiality: each can form any tissue or organ if properly signaled, but not a complete body.

Beyond the 16-cell stage, the fledging embryo, now called the blastocyst consisting of individual cells called blastomeres, begins to change drastically. In the accepted chronology, the cells on the outer surface begin transforming into a single layer of trophoblastic cells, the precursors of the placenta, while the more centrally located blastomeres give rise to the inner cell mass, destined to develop into the embryo body.[5;8;9]

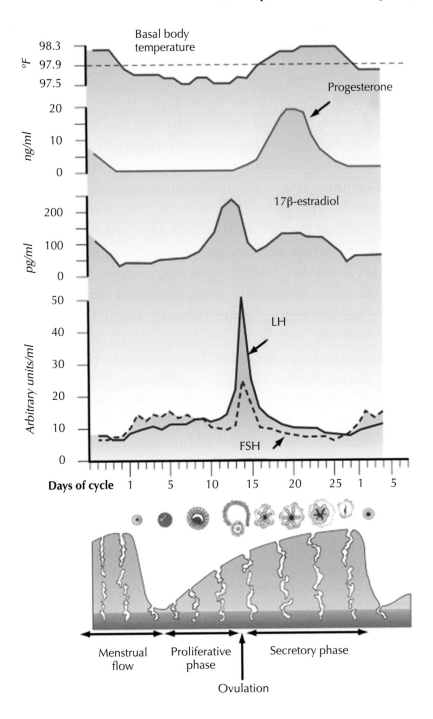

**FIGURE 4:** Levels of circulating gonadal and pituitary hormones
during the menstrual cycle.

*(Originally published in Carlson BM: Human Embryology & Developmental Biology,
4th Ed., St. Louis, Mosby, 2008. Copyright Mosby 2008. Used with permission.)*

As the blastocyst enters the uterine cavity, the trophoblasts begin secreting a group of trypsin-like proteolytic enzymes that digest away the zona pellucida, the outer protein shell. Now, six to seven days after conception, the growing blastocyst faces the daunting problem of implantation into the uterine lining, which requires active participation and mutual cooperation on the part of both the embryo and the endometrium. As Dr. Carlson writes:

> Successful implantation requires a high degree of preparation and coordination by both the embryo and the endometrium. The complex hormonal preparations of the endometrium that began at the close of the previous menstrual period are all aimed at providing a suitable cellular and nutritional environ-

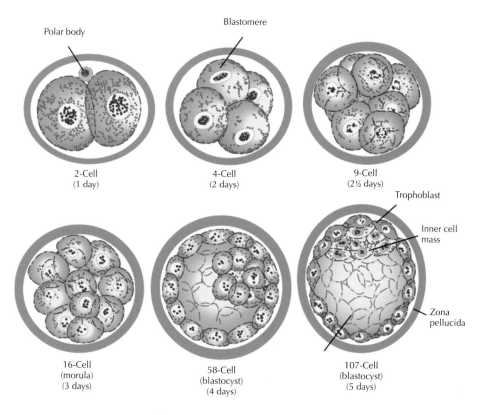

**FIGURE 5:** Early cleavage stages in the human embryo.

*(Originally published in Carlson BM: Human Embryology & Developmental Biology, 4th Ed., St. Louis, Mosby, 2008. Copyright Mosby 2008. Used with permission)*

ment for the embryo. Dissolution of the zona pellucida signals the readiness of the embryo to begin implantation.[4(p48)]

As it turns out the uterus can most effectively accept an egg between days 20 and 24 of the typical ovulatory cycle.[5] At other times, implantation simply will not succeed. During this brief period, as the blood supply to the uterine surface reaches a maximum, the endometrium itself becomes boggy, filled with nutritive fluids secreted by the uterine glands to help insure successful implantation of the embryo and its subsequent survival. At this point, on the luminal surface of each endometrial cell, microscopic cytoplasmic projections called pinopodes begin growing into the uterine cavity.[5] A dense coating of protein adhesion molecules of the integrin class coat each of these tiny membrane extensions, providing docking points for the trophoblast cells of the arriving embryo.[1;5] Many cell lines employ integrins to permit attachment to other cell types or to extracellular materials. For example, these proteins allow our various immune cells to adhere to areas of tissue debris after injury, to help begin the inflammation-repair process.

Once inside the uterus, the blastocyst must bond very quickly to the endometrial epithelium, if it is to survive. Usually, the embryo/trophoblast complex implants in the upper third of the uterine cavity, where a particularly rich network of integrin molecules on the epithelium provide convenient and efficient points of attachment.[4(p48)] In addition, the epithelial cells, under the direction of estrogen specifically, begin secreting a series of growth factors, including epidermal growth factor (EGF), that appear absolutely essential for successful implantation and survival of the embryo. Dr. Norwitz reports laboratory experiments with animals showing that if estrogen secretion is blocked as a fertilized egg approaches the endometrium, the epithelial cells fail to release epidermal growth factor, and the trophoblast will not adhere.[5]

In response to EGF, at the precise location where the blastocyst comes into contact with the endometrial lining, cells of the outer trophoblastic layer fuse together into syncytiotrophoblasts, giant cells with multiple nuclei embedded in a stream of shared cytoplasm (See Figure 6).[4(p52)] After this change, microvilli, small membrane projections coated with integrins, begin forming on the surface of the syncytiotrophoblast layer,

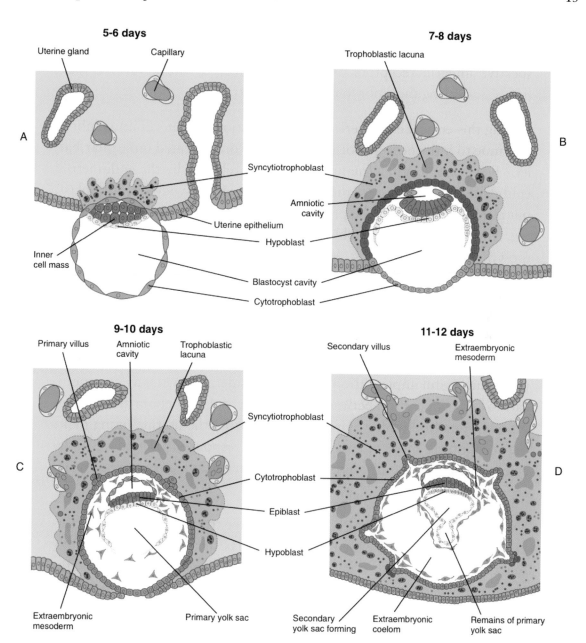

**FIGURE 6:** Major stages in implantation of a human embryo.

*(Originally published in Carlson BM: Human Embryology & Developmental Biology, 4th Ed., St. Louis, Mosby, 2008. Copyright Mosby 2008. Used with permission)*

directly opposite the pinopodes of the uterine epithelium. The trophoblastic microvilli intermingle closely with the pinopodes and the respective integrin receptors of each tissue merge, like keys in a lock, firmly anchoring the embryo to the endometrium.[5]

During this critical early period of implantation, the uterus and embryo continue to influence each other in a tightly orchestrated molecular ballet.[5] For example, epidermal growth factor released by the endometrial epithelium not only guides the development of the syncytiotrophoblast, but also directly signals the primitive embryonic cells to start proliferating. And in turn, the trophoblasts begin synthesizing a host of their own growth factors, including leukemia inhibiting factor, transforming growth factor alpha, transforming growth factor beta, platelet derived growth factor, insulin-like growth factor II, colony-stimulating factor 1, interleukin-1, and interleukin-6. These various peptides and proteins help make the uterine epithelium even more receptive to the embryonic tissues as they invade further into the deeper uterine layers.[5;10] At every point, successful implantation requires considerable two-way communication and cooperation between the endometrial epithelium and the embryo with its trophoblast. Growth factors from the uterine lining make the trophoblast more aggressive, while in response to signaling molecules released by the trophoblast, the epithelial lining more readily accepts invasion.[7]

Shortly after docking on the endometrium, the trophoblasts begin secreting various proteolytic enzymes of the matrix metalloproteinase family that can quite efficiently digest away type IV collagen and other proteins of the epithelial basement membrane, as well as the collagen glue of the underlying connective tissue.[5;6] Scientists recognize four classes of matrix metalloproteinases, altogether totaling more than 20 individual enzymes, each designed to attack a particular target molecule in the extracellular environment.[1;6]

As the various tissue barriers break down, the trophoblast can then migrate deep into the uterine tissue, bringing the embryo along with it. Dr. Carlson writes:

> Small projections of syncytiotrophoblast insert themselves between uterine epithelial cells. They then spread along the epi-

thelial surface of the basal lamina that underlines the endometrial epithelium . . . Within a day or so, syncytiotrophoblastic projections . . . begin to penetrate the basal lamina. The early syncytiotrophoblast is a highly invasive tissue, and it quickly expands and erodes its way into the endometrial stroma.[4(p52)]

During these early stages of adhesion and invasion, the trophoblastic cells begin secreting human chorionic gonadotropin (hCG), a hormone which, once absorbed into the maternal bloodstream, directly stimulates the corpus luteum of the ovary to continue releasing progesterone and estrogen.[4(p16);6] Without the stimulus of hCG, the corpus luteum deteriorates rapidly, so that both estrogen and progesterone levels fall to near zero. Without the requisite hormones present, the endometrial epithelium cannot efficiently synthesize the growth factors essential for successful implantation, and the whole process comes to a halt.

As the trophoblast penetrates deeper into the endometrium, the local epithelium converges around the blastocyst itself, so that by day 10–12 after conception, the embryo and its trophoblast lie completely imbedded within the uterine lining. At this point, progesterone synthesized by the maternal corpus luteum stimulates the embryonic cells to begin dividing even more rapidly, as the uterine stromal tissues form a dense capsule, the decidua, around the implanted blastocyst. This distinctive tissue not only manufactures nutritive substances such as glycogen to help feed the growing embryo, but also helps protects the embryo against attack by the various maternal immune cells present in the endometrial layers.[7]

Each of us carries in all our cells a unique genetic identity, unlike that of anyone else—unless we have an identical sibling—expressed on membrane surfaces as antigen proteins of the Major Histocompatibility Complex (MHC).[11] The pattern of these MHC molecules provides a fingerprint which helps our own immune system distinguish friendly cells from foe, that is, self from non-self. Normally, our lymphocytes, macrophages and neutrophils express the same exact membrane MHC proteins as all our other cell types. These shared antigens, this molecular commonality, signal the various immune cells that they are dealing with self, not foreign invaders. Should the MHC sequencing on a particular tissue differ from that of the immune defenders, the lymphocytes immediately go on the offensive, with possible deadly effect. As an example, we can reject a non-compatible organ transplant in an hour. In somewhat less dramatic fashion, in autoimmune diseases such as lupus, lymphocytes and other immune cells lose their ability to read MHC proteins properly, sensing self as foreign, with often disastrous results.[11]

The embryo and its trophoblast, with their own unique MHC fingerprint, differ genetically from the mother since half of their genes derive from the father. Despite the antigen incompatibilities that would normally provoke strong reactions, the embryonic tissues most commonly exist in a state of grace, safe from the potential menace of the mother's immunity. This situation seems particularly perplexing, since once the embryo implants, a variety of immune cells rapidly overrun the decidua, immediately adjacent to the growing embryo and its fledgling placenta. As Norwitz writes: "a minimum of 10 to 15 percent of all cells found in the decidua are lymphocytes."[5] Most are natural killer cells, usually the first cells to attack a foreign transplanted tissue, so the odds against the embryo and its trophoblast surviving would seem to be quite daunting. Surprisingly, the trophoblast itself, as it implants and invades, secretes a series of messenger chemokines, another class of peptides, into the blood supply of the mother. These in turn signal natural killer and other lymphocytes to aggregate right within the decidua, in close proximity to the genetically foreign trophoblast and embryo. In effect, our normally aggressive immune cells, our defenders against foreign invasion, come to the site of implantation because the trophoblast tells them to come.

The accumulation of natural killer and related cells, prompted by the trophoblast, resembles in detail the repair processes that occur in an area of tissue injury such as a skin wound. With any such damage, in response to chemokines released locally, large numbers of lymphocytes, monocyte-macrophages and neutrophils migrate to the site to guard against pathogenic microorganisms, to clear away debris, and to enhance tissue healing.[12;13(p703)] Of course, the implantation site within the uterus differs from a typical wound because here we don't want the foreign invader, the embryo, stopped, destroyed, and cleaned up. So, if this is the case, what benefit to the embryo would such an immune response serve? The answer lies in the process of angiogenesis—the growth of new blood vessels so critical to the survival of the embryo.

In its earliest stages, before the connections to the maternal circulation form, the embryo lives in a strongly hypoxic environment, since only small amounts of oxygen can diffuse through the uterine tissues.[7;14] At this point in its development, researchers suspect that higher oxygen levels might actually be harmful to the embryonic cells, allowing for the release of reactive oxygen species, the potentially destructive free radicals produced during normal metabolism.[7] These hyperactive molecules might easily disrupt biochemical processes within the blastomeres, even the embryonic DNA itself, provoking destructive or lethal mutations.

At some critical point, when diffusion no longer adequately supplies oxygen to the inner cells of the growing embryo, a steady vascular supply becomes essential for continued survival—hence the need for angiogenesis, and a stable connection to the maternal vasculature.

For the invading trophoblast/embryo complex, angiogenesis begins as the syncytiotrophoblastic cells migrate through the endometrium, ultimately reaching the maternal spiral arterioles and venules located in the underlying uterine stroma (See Figure 6-C and 6-D). At this point, a group of adhesion molecules normally localized on the endothelium, the cells that line the maternal vessels, begin appearing on the surface of the syncytiotrophoblasts, in a form of molecular mimicry. These shared surface proteins enable the migrating trophoblasts to begin penetrating into the small arteries and veins of the uterus to form the initial connections to the maternal blood supply.[5;6;10] At the same time, numerous endothelial cells begin migrating out of the vessel walls, creating small arterioles and venules that infiltrate into the trophoblastic tissue. With these vascular link-ups successfully established, the embryo can now access nutrients and oxygen from the mother, as well as rid itself of metabolic wastes.

The entire process requires the presence of growth factors such as vascular endothelial growth factor, which immune cells such as lymphocytes synthesize very efficiently.[1] In wound healing, lymphocytes in the area of injury release such angiogenic molecules to allow for new vessel growth, in turn guaranteeing a supply of nutrients and oxygen needed for tissue healing to proceed. In the decidua of the uterus, the large numbers of aggregating lymphocytes do the same, releasing signaling molecules that stimulate vessel formation, to provide the much needed blood supply into the trophoblastic tissues.

Nonetheless, surrounded by a large population of very active lymphocytes, particularly natural killer cells, the embryo and its trophoblast would seem to be at incredible risk of immunologic attack. After all, since an activated lymphocyte response can quickly and easily destroy a transplanted organ, a tiny embryo would hardly seem to be a difficult target. But the trophoblast quite effectively outsmarts the mother's defense mechanisms by suppressing its own MHC Class I and II proteins—those identified with tissue rejection—so that it seems invisible to maternal immune surveillance.[2]

The trophoblast also secretes a series of immune modulating molecules, such as the chemokine interleukin-10, that seem to disable the attack mechanism of these lymphocytes. Norwitz writes of one trophoblastic enzyme, indole-amine 2,3-dioxygenase, "that rapidly degrades tryptophan, which is essential for the activation of T cells [an aggressive subset of lymphocytes]."[5] In 2007, Lunghi reported that trophoblast signaling suppresses the aggressive T1 line of thymocytes, and instead stimulates the activity of the more quiescent T2 line.[7] As a result of such activity, the normally vigilant immune cells appear paralyzed, unable to move against the trophoblast, which thus adeptly usurps the maternal immune system, without any danger to itself. It signals lymphocytes, macrophages and neutrophils to congregate in the decidua to help with angiogenesis, while at the same time effectively blocking immune attack.

During the initial few weeks of pregnancy, as the trophoblastic tissues continue to invade, spreading in all directions, the connections between the embryo and the uterine blood supply become more complex (See Figure 7). Sprouts of the spiral arteries penetrate into the trophoblastic tissues to form lacunae in which maternal blood percolates.[4(p53);5;10] Blood vessels from the growing embryo also migrate deeply into the trophoblast, so that maternal and embryonic blood come into close physical contact, separated only by partitions, called villi, of trophoblastic cells. At this point, the trophoblast, now referred to as the chorion, resembles a sphere with the growing embryo inside and attached at one pole. Its cells, which appear far less amorphous than those of the earlier

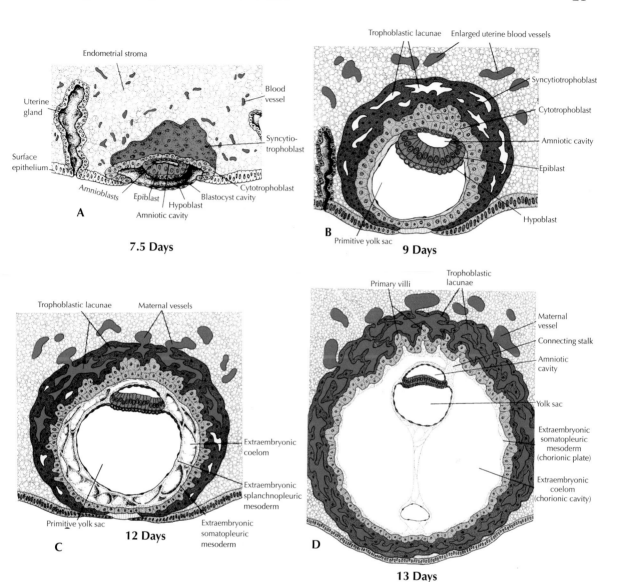

**FIGURE 7:** Development of vascular connections between the trophoblast and uterus.

*(Originally published in Sadler TW: Langman's Essential Medical Embryology, Baltimore, Lippincott Williams & Wilkins. Copyright Lippincott Williams & Wilkins 2005. Used with permission.)*

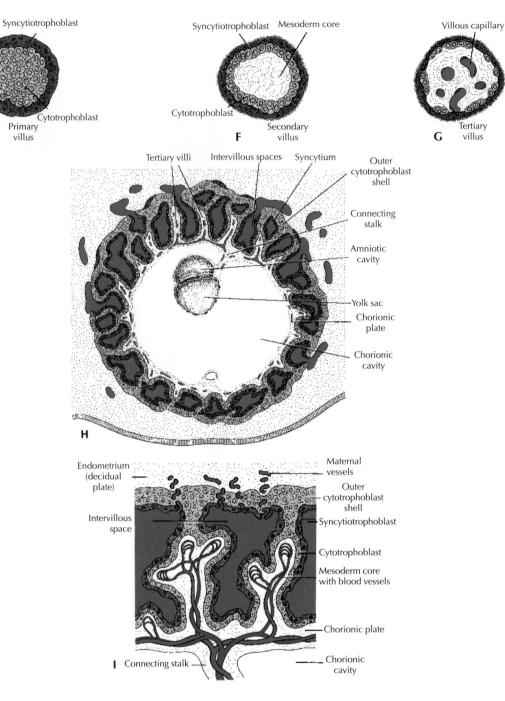

**FIGURE 7** *(continued)*

trophoblast, invade less aggressively. In reference to this change, Carlson writes:

> Trophoblastic processes enter the blood vessels [of the uterus] . . . By the time blood-filled lacunae have formed, the trophoblast changes character, and it is not as invasive as it was during the first few days of implantation.[4(p53)]

During weeks seven and eight after conception, the chorion tissues nearest to the embryo evolve into the mature placenta, while the more distant trophoblast cells undergo apoptosis, or programmed cell death. During this process, the surviving trophoblasts continue to change, appearing less and less amorphous, more and more differentiated, all the while behaving less aggressively. Eventually, as the placenta takes its final shape, invasion by the trophoblast cells ceases entirely.

As the trophoblast matures, the surrounding endometrium and decidua change markedly in their behavior as well. During the first weeks of pregnancy, endometrial and decidual cells release a host of growth and angiogenic factors that encourage the trophoblast to invade and migrate. With the embryo securely imbedded within the uterus, in a complete reversal the maternal cells begin secreting inhibitory molecules that *slow* invasion. Among these are a group of proteins that neutralize to some extent the matrix metalloproteinases, the enzymes needed by the trophoblast to digest away connective tissue obstacles and penetrate through the uterine wall. With its metalloproteinases inhibited, the trophoblast cannot continue migrating as aggressively through the underlying uterine layers.

Harvey J. Kliman, M.D., Ph.D., of the Yale University School of Medicine, makes the point that the endometrial cells themselves help moderate this change in trophoblast character from an aggressive to a more placid tissue:

> On the one hand trophoblasts have a potent invasive capacity and if allowed to invade unchecked, would spread throughout the uterus. The endometrium, on the other hand, controls trophoblast invasion by secreting locally acting factors (cytokines

and protease inhibitors), which modulate trophoblast invasion. Ultimately, normal implantation and placentation is a balance between regulatory gradients created by both the trophoblasts and endometrium.[15]

The highly differentiated tissues of the mature placenta resemble a circular disc, about 8–10 inches in diameter and 1–2 inches thick, weighing about a pound, lying firmly attached to the uterine decidua.[4] In its final incarnation, the placenta serves as a largely vascular organ with intricate interminglings between the maternal and fetal blood supplies (See Figure 8). Here, through complex processes of diffusion and active transport, the embryonic blood picks up all the nutrients and oxygen it needs from the mother's circulation, and releases carbon dioxide and other metabolic wastes for removal.

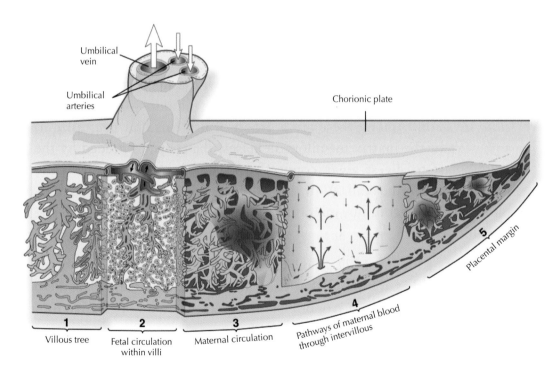

**FIGURE 8:** Structure and circulation of the mature human placenta.

*(Originally published in Carlson BM: Human Embryology & Developmental Biology, 4th Ed., St. Louis, Mosby, 2008. Copyright Mosby 2008. Used with permission.)*

Usually, this whole process of implantation, invasion, and placentation works efficiently, without a hitch. Most of the time, the trophoblast invades when it should invade, then matures on signal, its prodigious proliferative, invasive, migratory, and angiogenic activities gradually slowing to a halt. But not always; occasionally, if the trophoblastic cells fail to mature, instead remaining undifferentiated, proliferative, invasive, migratory, and angiogenic, gestational trophoblastic disease results.[16(p1297)]

This category of disorders usually is associated with a non-vital embryo—a sign perhaps that the living embryo itself, as it grows, helps regulate normal trophoblast behavior.[17] The term "gestational trophoblastic disease" actually refers to a range of distinct syndromes recognized even in Beard's day, from mild, benign conditions in which the trophoblast invades only locally to the aggressive life-threatening tumor choriocarcinoma.[16(p1297)] In this frank cancer, both cytotrophoblastic and syncytiotrophoblastic cells remain very aggressive, with the ability to metastasize quickly throughout the mother's body.

In summary, without the trophoblast, the embryo of any mammalian species, including our own, would not survive beyond fertilization. Trophoblastic cells can attach to, and invade into, the uterine epithelial lining; they synthesize human chorionic gonadotropin (hCG), which directs the maternal corpus luteum to continue its synthesis of progesterone, a hormone essential for uterine receptivity. The trophoblastic tissue furthermore kidnaps the mother's immune system, encouraging large numbers of lymphocytes and other immune cells to migrate into the uterine decidua in a mock inflammatory reaction, with the benefits of angiogenesis but without the problem of immune rejection. Then on cue, having done its job, this primitive undifferentiated tissue rather quickly changes character, behaving less aggressively, ultimately transforming into the mature, non-invasive placenta. Even if we disregard for a moment Beard's ideas about cancer as disordered trophoblast, this tissue would still be, in and of itself, quite an extraordinary one to consider.

# CHAPTER 2

# The Molecular Biology of the Trophoblast

For most of the past 100 years, since the days of Dr. Beard, embryologists generally have believed that the early trophoblast, ultimately destined to form the placenta, and the inner cell mass, the future embryo itself, developed simultaneously from the early blastocyst. Such has been the standard canon, but not everyone has accepted this traditional teaching. Dr. Beard, it seems always at odds with prevailing dogma, disagreed, claiming that the trophoblast actually formed *before* the inner cell mass. He proposed, based on his meticulous research of various embryonic specimens of various mammalian species, that not only did the trophoblast develop first, but that the inner cell mass, the future embryo, actually grew from the trophoblast as its direct offspring, in a sense making the trophoblast the ultimate parental tissue.[3]

In this regard, to Beard's great credit, recent advances now confirm what he reported, that the cells of the trophoblast appear *before* any other cell line. As Dr. James C. Cross at the University of California Medical Center, San Francisco, an expert on the molecular biology of the trophoblast, and his colleagues write:

> The first cell lineages to be established in the mammalian embryo contribute only to extraembryonic structures that form the placenta. It is only after implantation that significant differentiation occurs in the embryonic ectoderm, cells that give rise to all the structures of the embryo proper.[18]

Although the details remain to be worked out, we do know that early molecular signaling among the blastomeres themselves seems to *favor* the growth of the trophoblast and not the inner cell mass.[8]

In recent years, scientists such as Dr. Cross have begun to unravel the specific molecular systems that drive certain cells of the primitive blastocyst to become trophoblasts before the inner cell mass forms. Cross' group has isolated several nuclear proteins that appear key to this early embryonic metamorphosis, the most important of which consist of a series of helix-loop-helix (HLH) proteins, including Hxt, Oct-4, Mash-2, and Hand-1.[19;20] The term "helix-loop-helix" refers to their molecular structure, two spiral helixes looped together. Each of these transcription factors, as they are known, works directly on nuclear DNA, activating or repressing specific nucleic acid sequences that determine the fate of each blastomere during its earliest stages of growth.[21;22] Initially, certain HLH proteins guide the formation of the trophoblast; later, within the embryo body itself, these same molecules regulate the development of both nerve and muscle cells.[8]

One HLH protein, Hxt, becomes active before any distinctive tissues are evident, at a time the few cells present appear amorphous, totally indistinct, still retaining their totipotentiality.[18-20;23] At this juncture, in response to some outside as yet unidentified directive, certain blastocysts begin synthesizing Hxt, setting off in turn a host of reactions that transform the blastomere into a trophoblast. In its absence, the cell remains a blastomere. Cross reports that in one laboratory experiment, Hxt, when microinjected into mouse blastomeres whose ultimate fate, in terms of differentiation, had not yet been decided, always fueled the formation of trophoblasts.[18]

Another nuclear protein, Oct-4, has the exact opposite effect.[21;22] Initially, all blastocysts synthesize this molecule, but as Cross reports, in those cells destined to develop into trophoblasts, at some early point Oct-4 production shuts down completely. If injected into the early trophoblasts, the Oct-4 protein reverses the behavior of the cells, leaving them non-aggressive, unable to invade.[8]

The investigations of scientists like Dr. Cross show us just how and why the trophoblast appears before any other embryonic tissue. But, not only does the trophoblast arise initially, it seems to guide the development of the inner cell mass itself. For example, gastrulation, the formation of the three basic tissue lines in the embryo—known as the ectoderm, mesoderm and endoderm—begins right at the point where the inner cell mass connects to the overlying trophoblast; if that attachment should break, the trophoblast survives but the fledgling embryonic cells cease maturing and eventually die.[8] In this way, the trophoblast does more than simply invade into the uterus, it seems needed for embryonic growth itself.

In early development, such local influences between cells and tissues seem to be the rule.[24] For example, if cells from the inner cell mass, normally programmed to form the embryonic body, are transplanted to the outer cell layer, they transform into trophoblasts.[4(p45)] If early trophoblast cells are moved into the inner cell mass, they subsequently mature as normal embryonic body cells. These experiments illustrate that some very precise signals from the immediate molecular environment of these cells determine their future.

During the first weeks of embryogenesis, the primitive trophoblasts divide quickly, without much restraint. True, cells of the inner mass also replicate rapidly, but trophoblasts not only divide, they invade and migrate through the uterine tissue. Cells of the fledgling embryo can do neither on their own. This distinctive growth dynamic of the trophoblast, proliferation associated with invasion, seems under the control of yet another factor, the Mash-2 HLH. As blastocysts begin their transformation into trophoblasts, Mash-2 production turns on full bore, promoting both rapid cell division as well as invasive behavior. Without this particular factor present, the blastomeres remain non-aggressive. Mash-2, as Cross writes, "is expressed exclusively in proliferative trophoblast and that is required for maintenance of this pool of cells."[8]

While the trophoblast helps guide the formation of the inner cell mass, the influence works both ways. In the human embryo, eight weeks after conception only the trophoblastic cells in direct contact with the inner cell mass continue dividing rapidly while retaining their invasive potential.[8] It appears that molecular messages from the embryo, including epidermal growth factor, signal the nearby trophoblasts via membrane receptor pathways to continue their aggressive behavior. However, the bulk of the trophoblasts, those not adjacent to the embryo itself and away from the influence of its growth factors, change radically, both in appearance and behavior. They merge to form multinucleated giant cells, the syncytiotrophoblasts, that cease replicating and no longer invade.[4(p52);8]

In the syncytiotrophoblast, the change in character from an aggressive invasive tissue into dormancy seems regulated, within the cell nuclei, by a fourth helix-loop-helix protein, Hand-1. Unlike Hxt or Mash-2, both evident early in trophoblast history, Hand-1 doesn't appear until the trophoblasts located far from the inner cell mass begin merging.[20] At this point, as Hand-1 concentration increases, Mash-2 vanishes from the cells, in a type of mutual exclusivity—Mash-2 initially stimulating rapid growth and the invasive phenotype, Hand-1 later doing just the opposite, slowing trophoblast replication and pushing toward non-aggressive giant cell maturity.

In the early trophoblast, within the nucleus transcription factors such as Hxt and Mash-2 prod into action cyclin and cyclin-dependent kinase systems, enzymes that directly stimulate DNA to replicate and cells in turn to divide. Hand-1, in contrast, suppresses cyclin and cyclin dependent cascades, in effect inhibiting DNA replication and with it, cell division.

During the early stages of trophoblast life, when the cells divide rapidly and invade freely, they express three times the levels of cyclin B as when the cells become less invasive eight weeks after gestation. Then, as the trophoblast transforms into a collection of quiescent giant cells, the tumor suppressor gene p21, under the influence of Hand-1, synthesizes the p21 enzyme, which effectively suppresses the entire cyclin/cdkB system and consequently, cell replication.[25]

Finally, the proliferative, invasive, and migratory behavior of the early trophoblast always accompanies an undifferentiated phenotype, microscopically, a primitive, amorphous appearance of the cells, with an absence of distinguishing characteristics. As the trophoblast matures into the unique-looking giant syncytiotrophoblast line, and then ultimately into the placenta, the once rapidly dividing cells not only lose their pro-liferative and invasive potential, but dramatically change appearance.

Throughout embryonic development, this process of differentiation plays out, the gradual transformation of more primitive cells, both in terms of appearance and behavior, into the mature cell types of our various tissues and organs. Wikipedia actually provides about as good a definition of the process as we have seen:

> In developmental biology, **cellular differentiation** is the process by which a less specialized cell becomes a more specialized cell type. Differentiation occurs numerous times during the development of a multicellular organism as the organism changes from a single zygote to a complex system of tissues and cell types. . . . Cell differentiation causes its size, shape, polarity, metabolic activity, and responsiveness to signals to change dramatically. These changes are largely due to highly-controlled modifications in gene expression. With a few exceptions, cellular differentiation almost never involves a change in the DNA sequence itself. Thus, different cells can have very different physical characteristics despite having the same genome.[26]

As the primitive, amorphous blastocysts gradually transform into the 200 or so very distinctive tissues of the fully formed fetus, these embryonic cells change drastically, in terms of how they look, and how they act.[27(p510)] For example, mature neurons in an adult human, as a class, with their dendrites sprouting from one end and the thin axon at the other, their ability to transmit electro-chemical impulses, differ from elongated muscle cells containing actin and myosin filaments allowing for rapid contraction. Both nerve and muscle cells can be readily distinguished under the microscope from the columnar epithelium that line the intestinal mucosa, with their microvilli brush borders permitting the efficient absorption of nutrients. And the secretory cells of the exocrine pancreas, with their enzyme-filled vacuoles packed into the cytoplasm and their enormous protein synthesizing potential, bear little resemblance to nerve, muscle, or absorptive cells (See Figure 9).

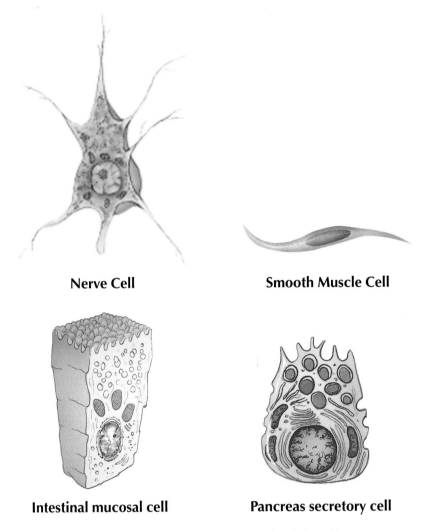

**Nerve Cell**                    **Smooth Muscle Cell**

**Intestinal mucosal cell**        **Pancreas secretory cell**

**FIGURE 9:** Different types of adult cells.

*(Originally published in Gartner LP and Hiatt JL: Color Atlas of Histology, 4th Ed., Baltimore, Lippincott Williams & Wilkins. Copyright Lippincott Williams & Wilkins 2006. Used with permission.)*

In maturity, each of these cell types looks completely different from the others, and performs completely different biochemical functions. Even within a particular tissue class, such as nerve, cells can vary enormously, structurally and behaviorally, depending on their particular responsibilities. The glia cells of the brain, the supportive neurons responsible for maintaining the myelin sheath, have only a slight resemblance to the preganglionic cells of the vagus, with their long axons extending from the brainstem to the upper intestinal tract. The differences, histologically and physiologically speaking, are indeed enormous.

Now, as we turn to the similarities between the early trophoblast and cancer, we will return to this process of differentiation, its absence in both cell lines, and its importance to our understanding of the unique behavior of each.

# CHAPTER 3

# Trophoblast Invasion, Migration, and Angiogenesis

The early trophoblast lacks differentiation in appearance, and specificity in function. Its cells appear primitive and indistinct; they proliferate initially without much restraint, invade adjacent tissues efficiently, and migrate easily through them before transforming into the mature, highly differentiated and non-aggressive placenta. Most of the time, the entire process of trophoblast implantation, growth and maturation proceeds flawlessly, though when control does falter, the very aggressive choriocarcinoma results. But choriocarcinoma occurs only rarely: usually the system works meticulously well.

Cancer cells, like trophoblasts, also lack differentiation in structure and in behavior; they too appear primitive, proliferate without restraint, invade without difficulty, and migrate through tissues easily. But cancer cells differ from trophoblast in that they never mature toward a differentiated phenotype, never shift behavior to a less aggressive form. Malignant cells, unless halted by effective treatment, will continue infiltrating local tissues and vessels, eventually metastasizing via the host's bloodstream or lymphatic channels to distant sites, where they migrate out of the vessels to begin the process of invasion anew. The pattern can be repeated in cancer, over and over again, until the patient ultimately dies.

Since their final destiny differs so dramatically, can the life history of the trophoblast teach us anything about why and how a cancer can invade and spread, so often with such unstoppable tenacity? Are there any real

connections between the ultimately controlled implantation of the trophoblast and the unrestrained invasion of cancer?

For the following discussion, we have relied on many sources, but most
heavily on the extraordinary work of Drs. Michael J. Murray and Bruce
A. Lessey, both of the Department of Obstetrics and Gynecology at
the University of North Carolina. In their 1999 article entitled "Embryo Implantation and Tumor Metastasis: Common Pathways of
Invasion and Angiogenesis," the two authors present one of the first
modern discussions linking with great precision the biology of the
trophoblast to the metastatic potential of cancer, in a way few scientists have since Dr. Beard.[1] In succeeding years others have followed
suit, including Ferretti and colleagues, focusing on the similarities, on
a molecular level, between the two cell lines, but the article by Murray and Lessey still provides a most perceptive review of the field.[2]

In the abstract of their article, Murray and Lessey say quite bluntly as
Beard himself implied so long ago, that cancer cells use *the very same
molecular techniques* for invasion employed by the trophoblast:

> Implantation of the embryo is one of the last great mysteries of re-
> productive biology. There are striking similarities present between
> the behavior of invasive placental cells and that of invasive cancer
> cells. In this review, we propose that cellular mechanisms used by
> the cells of the placenta during implantation are reused by cancer
> cells to invade and spread within the body. Integrins and other cell
> adhesion molecules, extracellular matrix and matrix metallopro-
> teinases all appear to be involved and are regulated by the complex
> endocrine . . . milieu within the uterus. Angiogenesis is a common
> feature of both implantation and cancer spread . . . An apprecia-
> tion of the maternal mechanisms to control this invasive behavior
> may likewise lead to a better understanding of metastatic cancer
> cells and lead to better methods to control their growth and spread
> within host tissues.[1]

As this brief paragraph shows, after 100 years, someone other than Dr.
Beard recognizes the "striking similarities" between the behavior of the
trophoblast and that of cancer. In the following sections, we will look at

these similarities in some detail, beginning by re-examining somewhat more closely the trophoblast as it infiltrates the uterus, then turning our attention to cancer and the mechanisms malignant cells use as they invade, migrate, and metastasize.

As we have seen, the process of implantation into the uterus begins with the attachment of the trophoblast to the epithelial cells of the endometrium, followed by the migration of the trophoblastic cells through this layer, and ultimately, their penetration into the underlying stromal tissues (See Figure 6, p. 15). Drs. Murray and Lessey sum up the process nicely:

> Beginning as a single cell, the fertilized egg rapidly divides and eventually the trophectoderm [trophoblast] invades, in a controlled and orderly fashion, interacting first with the epithelial and later the stromal and endothelial [blood vessel] components of the endometrium. It is easy to find similarities between this cardinal event in reproduction and the growth and spread of tumor cells in the setting of cancer.[1]

As aggressive a tissue as it may be, the trophoblast can anchor to the endometrium only between days 20–24 of the ovulatory cycle. Before or after this time slot, it simply fails to adhere, no matter how hard it might try. During this limited window of opportunity, it's not the trophoblast that undergoes some metamorphosis, rather it's the uterine lining that changes in a way that allows attachment to occur.

As Murray and Lessey write:

> Early in the secretory phase [day 1–14] the endometrial lining appears to represent a barrier to implantation . . . Embryos at this stage are capable of implanting almost anywhere in the body except the uterus and maintain all the intrinsic abilities to attach, migrate and invade . . . Thus, although embryos possess a capacity for invasion, the endometrium can both facilitate and limit this process.[1]

During the brief 4–5 day phase of optimal receptivity, large numbers of integrin receptors suddenly begin massing along the pinopodes on the surface of the epithelial cells lining the endometrium.[5] As we have seen, these proteins specifically *allow* the trophoblast-embryo complex to attach. Even a cell line as aggressive as the trophoblast simply can't penetrate into the uterine tissues without the cooperation of the endometrium and the presence of its integrin receptors.

Once safely in place, the trophoblast must now move through a series of formidable barriers, beginning with the cell-to-cell bonds known as the cadherins. These tough proteins glue the epithelial cells to one another quite firmly in "tight junctions," so named in deference to their strength.

Epithelial cells bond not only to each other, but also to the underlying basement membrane, another tough obstacle consisting of a fibrous cement of proteins and glycoproteins mingled together.[28] A tightly knit web of collagen, each molecule itself consisting of three strong protein fibers wrapped around one another in a triple helix, reinforces the basement membrane structure like a microscopic barbed wire. Along with the other basement membrane molecules, collagen creates a solid boundary between the epithelial cells above and the connective tissues below.

It would be difficult to overstate just how tough, on a molecular level, the epithelial barrier of the uterus, with its basement membrane, can be to an invader like the trophoblast. In fact, without the assistance of the epithelium itself, the trophoblast could not penetrate any further, but once the endometrial cells have *permitted* the trophoblast to attach, the epithelial cells themselves set the stage for subsequent invasion.[1;10]

During the brief period when the endometrium is receptive, the specific integrin receptors a1b1 for collagen and laminin, the a4b1 receptor for fibronectin, and the avb3 integrin for vitronectin sprout in large numbers on the epithelial cell surfaces.[1] This precise pattern of integrins helps the embryo to attach, and with the connections established, these same three integrins begin appearing on the trophoblast cell surfaces, in a type of molecular mirroring. The trophoblast essentially mimics the uterine epithelium, and for good reason: this shared integrin pattern allows its cells to move more easily through the endometrium. Apparently, the uterine cells, now perceiving the invading trophoblasts as more of their own, in response loosen their tight junctions.

As the trophoblast-embryo complex moves more securely into the uterine lining, the epithelium begins releasing several growth factors that quickly bind to receptors on the trophoblast membranes. Once attached, these ligands, as such signaling molecules are called, turn on transduction cascades within the trophoblasts that on the very level of the DNA modify cellular behavior toward a more invasive phenotype.

In these signaling systems, a very active topic in cancer research, a ligand such as a neurotransmitter, peptide, or hormone attaches to a membrane receptor which, now activated, behaves as an enzyme within the cell membrane and within the underlying cytoplasm. For example, in the much studied tyrosine kinase cascade, when an appropriate ligand such as insulin binds at the cell surface, the receptor responds by phosphorylating itself, that is, adding a phosphate group, an event that essentially turns the complex into a vital enzyme. This phosphorylated ligand-receptor complex then sets off a series of cytoplasmic reactions which, depending on the circumstance, can either stimulate or suppress cell responses, including DNA transcription.[29(pp31-40)]

Within the trophoblast, a series of such molecular messages ultimately prompts its DNA to orchestrate the synthesis of matrix metalloproteinases (MMP), primarily MMP-2 and MMP-9.[1;2;10] The "metallo" in the term metalloproteinases refers to the metal zinc contained in all members of the group, the term proteinases indicates their objective, the efficient digestion of proteins.

Trophoblasts secrete their metalloproteinases into the uterine epithelium in an inactive precursor form, but on cue the cells release a second set of proteases that transform each proenzyme into its active conformation. These viable metalloproteinases in turn quickly digest away the cadherin bonds between epithelial cells, before attacking the underlying basement membrane, where they degrade type IV collagen as well as the denatured form of collagen known as gelatin.[1;2]

The trophoblast cells can now freely migrate through these breaks in the epithelial lining, only to face the next major hurdle, the stromal layer of the uterus, the connective tissue that lies underneath and supports the endometrium. Far thicker than the epithelial layer, this region provides a very effective tissue barrier, consisting of dense fibrous molecules such as fibronectin, laminin, vitronectin and collagen, all coiled around each other like layer after layer of tightly bound cords. Fibroblasts dispersed throughout the stroma secrete these various molecules into the extracellular matrix (ECM), which also serves as a support for the small uterine blood vessels, both arterioles and venules.

The trophoblasts begin attacking this obstacle again using the matrix metalloproteinases, named for their ability to digest the extracellular matrix, the ground substance of the stromal tissues. The enzymes perform the task quite efficiently, allowing the embryo and its trophoblast to invade into the deeper stromal tissues; there, the trophoblast anchors close to the uterine spiral arteries, whose blood supply will allow for continued growth.

Cells other than trophoblasts also secrete matrix metalloproteinases during the invasion process, including the stromal fibroblasts themselves, in response to growth factors released by the trophoblasts.[1] Once again, the uterine cells act to help the trophoblast move through another potentially daunting barrier.

This cooperation between trophoblast and uterus goes a step further. Extracellular matrix proteins such as fibronectin and laminin serve as more than biological glue holding the stromal layers together. Like all proteins, the ECM molecules consist of chains of amino acids, arranged in a specific sequence. The metalloproteinases cleave these matrix components at precise amino positions, leaving small peptide fragments with their own considerable biological activity, not apparent in the intact protein. Some of these peptides function as growth factors; others, including one small part of the laminin molecule, act as chemotactic agents, attracting trophoblast cells still deeper into the stroma. Others signal the trophoblast itself to release still more MMPs, needed to continue the digestion of the ECM. It appears that the trophoblast can invade deeply only in the presence of these matrix fragments; so, as the trophoblastic enzymes digest the extracellular matrix, the ECM fragments help move the trophoblast along.

Researchers refer to this intricate cooperation between cells in a tissue and the ECM peptides as "dynamic reciprocity," nicely described by

Drs. Murray and Lessey. Although the process isn't limited to trophoblast invasion, it certainly applies to it:

> The activities of MMPs include the regulation of cellular function through modification of the surrounding ECM. The term 'dynamic reciprocity,' coined by Bissell, refers to the concept that a cell synthesizes and secretes the ECM and is then altered by this ECM through specific receptors on its cell surface. The signal generated by this interaction is complex and can modify cellular phenotype including cell shape and gene expression.[1]

These extracellular matrix fragments perform their assigned tasks by attaching to integrin receptors on the trophoblast membrane. Integrins, as we have seen, localize on the surfaces of a number of different cell types during implantation, including the epithelial and stromal cells of the uterus, as well as on the trophoblast. Researchers have already isolated some 22 different integrin receptors, each of which, when activated by ligand, sets off precise transduction signaling cascades. As Drs. Stetler-Stevenson and Kleiner concisely write:

> Considerable redundancy within cell-ECM interaction mediated by integrins exist, because most integrins bind to several individual matrix proteins, and ECM components, such as laminin, fibronectin, vitronectin, and collagens, bind to several different integrin receptors. This fact suggests that integrins are capable of providing the cell with detailed information about the surrounding ECM environment, which is then integrated at the cellular level to generate a cellular response.[29(p129)]

As invasion continues, these ECM fragments seem to regulate trophoblast behavior very subtly, on many levels. For example, the metalloproteinases very efficiently digest away the underling uterine matrix, allowing for continued migration. However, if unchecked, this intense enzymatic activity could essentially dissolve the connective tissue to the point that the uterus simply would fall apart, hardly a desirable outcome. To prevent such a catastrophe, in response to another set of ECM fragments appearing late in the process, invading trophoblasts along with the stromal fibroblasts begin jointly secreting a series of metalloproteinase *inhibitors* that ward off excessive stromal digestion. During trophoblast invasion, remodeling of the extracellular matrix is thus very tightly controlled, to allow infiltration without total tissue destruction.[1;2;10]

Once imbedded in the stroma, the trophoblast must overcome one final obstacle, the critical need for an adequate blood supply. As the trophoblast penetrates through the epithelium and the underlying tissue barriers, the embryo itself grows rapidly, in turn requiring an increasing supply of nutrients and oxygen. Initially sufficient quantities of these essentials diffuse from local maternal vessels through the uterine stroma to sustain the embryo. Beyond a certain point, the embryo can't survive without direct access to the mother's circulation, which provides nutrients and oxygen and removes metabolic wastes.[30]

The trophoblast overcomes this obstacle adeptly; the same matrix metalloproteinases that helped forge a pathway through the endometrium and underlying connective tissue permit invasion into the walls of small stromal arteries and veins, the first step toward accessing the maternal blood supply.[1] But the trophoblast uses even more subtle tools than these digestive enzymes, to establish the much needed vascular connections. By this point, the integrins a1b1 and a4b1, dispersed as they are on the trophoblast cell membranes, have allowed it to slip through the epithelial lining. Now in response to signals from the trophoblasts, this same group of integrins begins appearing on the surface of the endothelial cells lining the local uterine blood vessels. This shared pattern of receptors allows the trophoblasts to move more easily into the vessel walls and into the inner endothelial lining, whose cells perceive these invaders as their kin. The migrating trophoblasts quickly establish themselves, setting the stage for the next step, when newly forming arterioles and venules from the embryo grow toward and intermingle with the maternal vasculature.[8;30]

As the trophoblasts make their way into the local vessels, the maternal immune cells, including lymphocytes and macrophages aggregating in the uterine stroma, begin secreting vascular endothelial growth factor (VEGF). At the same time, the trophoblasts start synthesizing two similar molecules, fibroblast growth factor (FGF) and placental growth factor (PGF). All three serve as angiogenic signals that help complete the connections between the embryonic and maternal blood supplies.[1;8]

Under the influence of VEGF, FGF and PGF, the normally quiescent endothelial cells begin proliferating rapidly themselves, and turn invasive. Using tools such as their own matrix metalloproteinases and integrin receptors, these cells migrate from their protected niche in the spiral arterioles and venules to make their way through the dense extracellular matrix, creating small vessels as they go. Eventually, the developing arteries and veins connect with the circulatory system of the embryo to provide for its growing metabolic needs.

Before these connections form, embryonic growth proceeds quite slowly, impeded by an hypoxic environment. With a steady source of nutrients and oxygen now available, growth takes off in an exponential fashion, as Drs. Murray and Lessey report:

> Embryos remain viable both in vitro [in the test tube] and in utero before implantation with minimal change in size. After trophoblast invasion and embryo neovascularization occur with communication to the maternal blood supply, embryos exhibit a logarithmic growth phase, *reminiscent of that seen in tumors* [italics ours].[1]

The successful implantation and survival of the embryo involve precise coordination between the trophoblast and uterine cells. Now having hopefully made this point, we would like to turn to the subject of cancer, which in terms of its invasive potential really doesn't differ much from the early trophoblast. Though we tend to think of malignancy in destructive and deadly terms, surprisingly enough its capacity to invade, in fact its very survival, requires a very similar cooperation between the tumor cells and the host tissues. A cancer, to flourish, cannot make it on its own; it needs help, which too often it gets.

It would be of benefit to review several basic points about the disease, before we move on. Approximately 90% of malignancies, including the major killers such as lung, colorectal, breast, pancreatic and prostate cancer, develop in epithelial tissues, the tissues lining our various organs and glands.[31] Such cancers fall into the category of carcinomas, which differ from sarcomas arising in connective tissues, such as in the stroma of an organ or in muscle. Malignancies we associate with the blood and lymph system—Hodgkin's disease, the leukemias, lymphomas, and myeloma, for example—form from immune cell precursors. But whatever the type or the site of origin, all cancer cells invade efficiently, with the capacity to infiltrate normal tissues aggressively and metastasize to distant sites.

The growth and subsequent spread of the epithelial cancers, the most common of malignancies, most closely approximates the trophoblast as it penetrates the uterine lining.[1,2] But the discussion that follows applies in a general sense to the mechanisms all cancers use, as they proliferate, invade, and metastasize.

Now, as we begin our foray into the biology of cancer, we would like to quote from the article of Drs. Murray and Lessey, in which they emphasize the similarities in behavior between trophoblast and malignancy:

> Tumor cells have borrowed many of the mechanisms for invasion used by the trophoblast to intrude into host tissues and establish their blood supply . . . Cellular gene expression first used during embryonic implantation and evolved mechanisms of invasion employed by the trophoblast are commonly used by cancer cells as they spread and invade the host tissues.[1]

An epithelial cancer cell, wherever it arises, faces the same obstacles as the embryonic trophoblast, with one exception. A malignant cell forming in an epithelium of an organ has no need to attach as does a trophoblast arriving in the uterine cavity, since it develops right there, within the tissue itself. But a newly formed cancer must nonetheless navigate through the cadherin connections between epithelial cells, the underlying tough basement membrane and the even tougher and denser extracellular matrix of the stroma. These barriers exist not only in the endometrium of the uterus, but in one way or another, in all our organs.

Normal epithelial cells, in whatever tissue they might live, always attach tightly to one another through the cadherin proteins on their membrane surfaces. These bonds form tight junctions that not only anchor the cells in place, but impede any invading threat, be it trophoblast, infectious micro-organism, or cancer. Malignant cells lack such bonds themselves, so consequently have a freedom of movement not seen in healthy epithelium. In fact researchers generally describe as one of the first steps in the formation of an epithelial cancer the "loss" of these tight junctions. Should these attachments remain in place, any cell, even a cancer cell, goes nowhere.

Drs. Stetler-Stevenson and Kleiner, writing in *Cancer: Principles & Practice of Oncology*, make clear the point that close connections between cells are incompatible with full blown cancer:

> The initial events in cellular invasion are changes in cell adhesion
> . . . Tumor cells must decrease cell and matrix adhesive interactions to escape . . . [29(p127)]

As a cancer begins its invasion into an organ, the cadherin attachments, these tight junctions between the normal epithelial cells, represent the first barrier it must cross. To help break through this obstacle, tumor cells secrete the same series of matrix metalloproteinases used by the trophoblast during its journey through the endometrium. In whatever tissue the cancer may be, the enzymes digest away the cadherin bonds rapidly and efficiently.

As Stetler-Stevenson and Kleiner write:

> Yet another mechanism to alter E[epithelial]-cadherin function is proteolytic modification. Lochter et al. have reported that E-cadherin function can be disrupted by degradation of E-cadherin's extracellular domains by stromelysin-1, a member of the matrix metalloproteinase (MMP) family that has been closely linked with tumor progression. [29(p127)]

Once successfully past the cadherin barrier, cancer cells then face the basement membrane, with its tough protein cords and encoiled collagen chains. To a pathologist, migration through the epithelial basement membrane signals one of the defining events in cancer formation.

Benign epithelial tumors such as fibrocystic breast lesions, no matter how big they grow, do not and cannot penetrate into or beyond the basement membrane.[13(p453);16(p154)] Only a few cell types, such as the trophoblast and the cells of cancer, seem able to do this.

Like the trophoblast, a growing malignancy cannot pass through this barrier on its own, it needs the help of the basement membrane to guide it on its way. After the cadherin junctions have been disrupted, integrin receptors on the surface of the cancer cells adhere to specific amino acid sequences of the basement membrane proteins, much as pieces of a puzzle fit together. Once activated, the receptors then turn on transduction pathways within the cancer cell that signal for a surge in matrix metalloproteinase synthesis. When released into the nearby environment, these enzymes efficiently digest away openings in the otherwise tough basement membrane, a process described by Drs. Stetler-Stevenson and Kleiner:

> Tumor cell interaction with the basement membrane is defined as the critical event of tumor invasion that signals the initiation of the metastatic cascade . . . Early studies on defining the invasive phenotype on malignant tumor cells focused on the interaction of tumor cells with the epithelial basement membrane. These studies defined the three-step hypothesis of tumor cell invasion: tumor cell attachment to the basement membrane, creation of proteolytic defects in the basement membrane, and migration of tumor cells through these defects.[29(p127)]

With the basement membrane breached, cancer cells can quickly pour through into the underlying connective tissue stroma. Here, in the dense, fibrous matrix, tumor cells could easily become bogged down, but the matrix metalloproteinases enable them to make headway as in the case of the trophoblast penetrating the uterus. But even with these potent enzymes at their disposal, cancer cells—like the trophoblast—cannot travel very far into the stroma without the direct cooperation of the extracellular matrix. The enzymes released from the invading malignancy, no matter how strong they may be, aren't sufficient to get the job done. So, to move the process along, as the cancer cells slowly migrate deeper into the extracellular matrix, stromal cells, including fibroblasts and immune cells—which we usually think should be *protecting* us—begin secreting large amounts of their own metalloproteinases. Surprisingly, our own normal cells, including our normal *immune* cells, not only assist the invading cancer, but are absolutely necessary for the invasion to continue. Some evidence indicates that the healthy stromal cells release more of the MMPs during the process than do the malignant cells themselves![1]

The cooperation between the cancer cells and the stromal components, for the benefit of the invading malignancy, involves more than the secretion of the MMPs. As in the case of the trophoblast, these enzymes cleave the various ECM proteins such as collagen, fibronectin, and laminin into smaller peptides that themselves can act as growth and chemotactic factors. And as the tumor cells migrate deeper into and through the stroma, integrin receptors start sprouting on their membrane surface that can bond to the ECM fragments. Working again through transduction pathways, a number of these peptides signal the cancer cells to continue dividing; others direct the tumor to continue invading.

On their membranes, invading cancer cells express the very same integrin receptors for these ECM fragments found on the trophoblast surface, as it penetrates the uterus. As Drs. Murray and Lessey, in discussing an experimental laboratory model of melanoma, write:

> Melanoma appears to be an excellent model for studying the invasive phenotype of cancer cells. Up-regulation of the vitronectin [an ECM protein] receptor, avb3, is clearly associated with the acquisition of an invasive and metastatic phenotype . . . This pattern of integrin expression is virtually identical to that noted for invasive cytotrophoblasts as they acquire the ability to invade the maternal vasculature.[1]

At this point, with the cancer cells moving through, stromal fibroblasts begin secreting another group of growth factors, including insulin-like growth factor, that signal for even more aggressive cell division and more aggressive penetration—just as the uterine fibroblasts assist the trophoblast.

But as in the case of the trophoblast, MMP activity must be tightly regulated for cancer invasion ultimately to succeed. With too much digestion, with too much of the extracellular matrix destroyed, the tissue would literally fall apart, along with the cancer. It is of no benefit to a spreading tumor if the ECM turns into an amorphous soup, with nothing to move through or anchor to. In such a situation, the cancer cells, along with all other stromal cells, would simply die. The malignant cells themselves—just like the trophoblast—avoid such an outcome by releasing, as their penetration advances, inhibitors of the MMP enzymes, so that the breakdown of the stroma and the ECM proceeds sufficiently to allow migration without total tissue annihilation. This coordination between MMP action and inhibition must be very precise.

Drs. Stetler-Stevenson and Kleiner make this point:

> Although these experiments and many others like them have demonstrated the key role of matrixin[MMP]-initiated degradation in tumor invasion and metastasis, the role of these enzymes in this process is more complicated than an [sic] 'degradation equals invasion" paradigm would suggest. Uninhibited matrix degradation would lead to complete dissolution of matrix proteins and would prevent tumor cells from being able to form attachments to each other or to matrix proteins, which is a necessary part of the tumor invasion mechanism. Thus, there is an implied balance between active proteases and inhibitors that results in an optimal invasive phenotype.[29(p134)]

At all levels, the cooperation between invading tumor and host resembles very closely what happens as the trophoblast makes its way through the uterine lining and underlying tissues. As Drs. Murray and Lessey write:

> Studies support the notion that ECM may provide signal transduction important in establishing the invasive phenotype. Once invasion has begun, the degradation products of ECM components such as laminin may stimulate migration and further the establishment of the invasive phenotype. Molecules made

by the surrounding parenchyma may, in some cases, influence the potential of either cancer cells *or trophoblast* [italics ours] to invade.[1]

Once established in the stroma, an invading cancer, just like the trophoblast, requires a steady and substantial blood supply in order to continue growing. Researchers estimate that a fledgling tumor cannot expand beyond one cubic millimeter in size without a direct connection to the host vasculature, so the formation of new vessels must be an essential next step.[1] For this process, a malignancy uses precisely the same tools as the trophoblast.

First, as the tumor enlarges, the cells on the leading edge begin sprouting the very same integrin receptors found on the endothelium of the host's normal small arteries and veins, in an analogous fashion to the angiogenic processes of the trophoblast. This mimicry permits the cancer cells, now masquerading as endothelium, to move easily right into the vessel walls.

Drs. Murray and Lessey describe this process, again using melanoma as an example:

> As reviewed earlier, human cytotrophoblasts and invasive melanoma exhibit similar patterns of integrin expression that have been shown to adopt a vascular phenotype capable of invading maternal spiral arterioles, strikingly similar to those noted in endothelial cells as they migrate toward the tumor.[1]

In addition, as the cancer invades, stromal immune cells, including lymphocytes and macrophages, secrete the same series of angiogenic factors, including vascular endothelial growth factor (VEGF), released during trophoblast migration. The tumor cells, like trophoblast cells, in response release fibroblast growth factor (FGF). Both VEGF and FGF signal the endothelial cells of the host, through integrin receptors on their surfaces and signal transduction, to turn invasive. Using their own matrix metalloproteinases, these vessel cells leave their home base, migrating through the ECM toward the tumor, creating small blood vessels along the way—just as they do during trophoblastic angiogenesis.[1]

In an expanding cancer, cell replication initially proceeds relatively steadily, though slowly. Once the newly forming vessels connect to the tumor, allowing for a rich supply of nutrients and oxygen, proliferation soars exponentially, just as it does when the maternal arterioles and venules reach the embryo during fetal growth. Drs. Murray and Lessey report that the volume of a tumor can increase *16,000 times* once the vascular connections become operational.[1] And with angiogenesis successfully established, a malignancy can then send seedling cells through the host's bloodstream, where at distant sites, and in other organs, they can attach to normal tissues (ironically, just as the trophoblast initially implants into the uterus). Then, the whole process of invasion, migration, and angiogenesis follows, and can be repeated, again and again until death ultimately ensues.

Without such intricate molecular coordination and cooperation with the host, cancer cells go nowhere, just as the trophoblast would go nowhere. We can of course understand these interactions in the case of the early placenta, but with deadly cancer, such synergism certainly seems counterproductive. Why would our normal tissues work so hard to help a tumor survive, grow, and invade? This molecular scenario makes no sense—it makes no sense, that is, unless the epithelial cells and stromal tissues have been fooled into thinking that tumor invasion is a good thing happening, a normal healthy process. Why else would they cooperate? Perhaps in all epithelial tissues, in whatever organ they may be, a genetic memory remains that, with certain molecular signals, provokes them into behaving like the receptive endometrium receiving an embryo. Such a proposal seems hardly far-fetched, since all epithelial tissues resemble one another to some extent in the way they look and in the way they behave, biochemically and genetically.[16(p142)] In both men and women, many epithelial cells, even in such organs as the pancreas and the intestines, express on their membrane surfaces estrogen receptors, and seem just like the endometrium to require, at least to some degree, such steroid hormone input for their normal growth and development. Maybe all epithelial tissues, when faced with a cell gone awry, respond with some deep-seated molecular reflex that makes them accept and aid the tumor.

Drs. Murray and Lessey, with no apparent knowledge of Dr. Beard's work, bring us to their conclusion that cancer, in its behavior, in its molecular biology, is just *like* the trophoblast:

> Tumors employ many of the same methods to grow and spread as first used by the cytotrophoblast. Tumor invasion and embryo implantation share common features. Like the trophoblast, tumor cells migrate through and invade their surrounding ECM. Access to vasculature and an ability to recruit a blood supply are also hallmarks of tumors and early embryos, needed to achieve exponential growth patterns that would be otherwise unattainable. There is much to be learned about these shared cellular protocols. Advances toward understanding both embryo and tumor invasion and angiogenesis will facilitate the discovery of methods for disrupting tumor growth and neovascularization. Such advances are likely to provide significant clinical benefit.[1]

# CHAPTER 4

# The Trophoblast *Is* Cancer

With its undifferentiated histology, in its aggressive potential, its capacity for invasion, migration, and angiogenesis, the trophoblast serves as an ideal model for cancer behavior. Contemporary scientists such as Ferretti et al, and Murray and Lessey make this point well. But Beard, in his research and writings went a step further, beyond the trophoblast as the perfect biological analogy for the behavior of malignant tissues; he insisted that cancer, whatever the type or form, develops *only* from misplaced trophoblastic cells, leftovers from our earliest embryonic past. In the Beardian cosmology, cancer is trophoblast, and always trophoblast.

Beard reached this conclusion as a result of his study of germ cells, the precursors to the adult gametes—eggs in the female ovaries, sperm in the male testes. The word "germ" in this case refers not to infectious micro-organisms, but rather to its technical meaning in embryology as those cells that ultimately, in the adult, give rise to the gametes. Scientists differentiate germ cells from what they call somatic cells, those that make up the various tissues and organs of a complex organism (other, that is, than the gamete precursors).

And indeed, the germ cell line does have a unique history, embryologically speaking, compared to any other body tissue. Researchers now know that by day 6, as implantation begins, the embryo consists of over 100 cells, including those of the outer trophoblast, at this point a sac-like lining one cell thick positioned around the growing spheroid blastocyst. The cells of the inner cell mass, the future embryo body, then aggregate at one pole of the trophoblast, while fluid fills the remainder of the blastocyst cavity.

Just as the trophoblast begins to implant, two distinct cell lines emerge from the inner cell mass, an upper layer, or epiblast, and a lower layer, known as the hypoblast.[4(p61)] The epiblast, as it matures, eventually gives rise to the embryo body proper, while the hypoblast develops into a set of extraembryonic structures. In birds and reptiles, the hypoblast forms the large yolk of the egg, which provides the essential nourishment for the

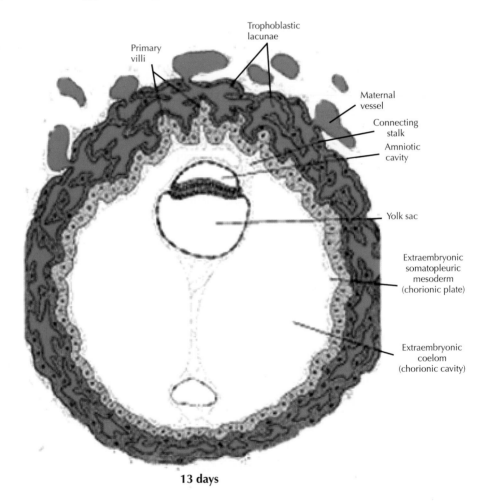

**13 days**

**FIGURE 10:** The early yolk sac in the human.

*(Originally published in Sadler TW: Langman's Essential Medical Embryology,*
*Baltimore, Lippincott Williams & Wilkins.*
*Copyright Lippincott Williams & Wilkins 2005. Used with permission.)*

embryo. Mammals, with their placental attachments in place, have no need for such a source of nutrients, so not surprisingly the yolk sac never matures beyond a primitive entity located outside the embryo body at the base of the developing umbilical cord (See Figure 10). Though this tissue remains relatively small throughout embryonic life, it still serves a critical function first observed by Beard a century ago.

We know from studies in mice that as the two tissue lines differentiate from the inner cell mass, a small group of primordial germ cells appears at the posterior end of the epiblast (See Figure 11). Over the next few days, these cells migrate en masse away from the epiblast and the future embryonic body to the posterior wall of the yolk sac located at the base of the future umbilical cord, quite a distance to travel, in cellular terms, from the developing embryo.[32] Of all fetal tissues, only the germ cells develop in this way, at some distance from the body proper; the precursors for all other adult tissues never leave the vicinity of the epiblast from which they arise.[4(p61);32]

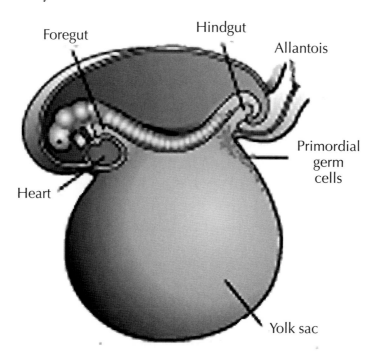

**FIGURE 11:** Primordial germ cells on the yolk sac.

*(Originally published in Sadler TW: Langman's Essential Medical Embryology, Baltimore, Lippincott Williams & Wilkins. Copyright Lippincott Williams & Wilkins 2005. Used with permission.)*

In humans, the primordial germ cells appear in the yolk sac by day 24 after fertilization where, in this nurturing environment—but outside and at a distance from the embryo itself—they begin dividing rapidly.[4(p2,p376)] During this fourth week of development, a number of these primitive germ cells emerge from the posterior yolk sac wall to begin migrating back toward the embryo body. In mice, about 100 germ cells set off on this trek that, beyond the yolk sac, follows a circuitous path through the stalk of the growing umbilical cord to the embryo itself. There the germ cells gather at the opening of the hindgut, the tissue that eventually forms the lower segments of the intestinal tract. The cells then enter the embryo itself, where they continue their journey through the complex tissues of the developing digestive system until they reach the genital ridge, the region destined to give rise to the adult gonads. At this point, the germ cells incorporate themselves into the maturing gonadal tissues.[4(p2, p376)]

During this circular trip, the germ cells propel themselves with ameboid movements along what appear to be predetermined pathways, laid out with specific biochemical signposts. One signaling system may involve integrin proteins on the surface of the germ cells, the same class of proteins that allows the trophoblast to attach to the uterine lining. During their migration, the integrin molecules enable the germ cells to pull themselves along by attaching to the connective tissue components of the embryo.[32] And as the cells travel through the hindgut tissues, they proliferate in response to growth factors secreted into the local microenvironment. By the time they reach their destination at the genital ridge, these cells will each have gone through six or seven divisions, yielding some 4000 offspring.[4(p2)]

In his text, Carlson describes an interesting experiment that shows just how powerful the homing instinct of the primordial germ cells can be. If the hindgut tissues of a mouse embryo containing germ cells in transit are transplanted into a different region of the gut, far removed from the normal pathways, the cells will still be found sometime later moving toward the genital ridge.[4(p377)]

Under normal circumstances, not all germ cells successfully complete the journey. The trip from the epiblast to the posterior wall of the yolk sac, back to the embryo then through the embryo itself to the genital ridge, involves movement through long distances, molecularly speaking, and requires precise signaling between the germ cells and the embryonic tissues. It is a difficult undertaking, so it is not surprising that hundreds essentially lose their way, ending up in a variety of non-gonadal tissues such as the intestines and the chest organs. Many of these wayward cells die, but many survive for the life span of the organism, hidden away wherever they might have come to rest.

Beard, among his many accomplishments in more conventional embryology, first described in some detail the maturing of germ cells early during development, and their peculiar journey from the epiblast to the yolk sac and back to the embryo body, observations that have held up with the passage of time. But he also, 100 years ago, first reported the existence of what he called "vagrant" germ cells, those which fail to complete the journey to the genital ridge, as a result of his studies of the Elasmobranch fish, a group including sharks, skates, and rays. As he writes in his book *The Enzyme Treatment of Cancer*:

> The number of Elasmobranch embryos hitherto examined is several hundred, belonging to different species, and in all these under a certain age no single embryo has been seen, in which all the germ-cells present might be described as normally placed. The percentage of vagrant germ-cells varies; it is usually from 10 to 12 per cent. in *Pristiurus*, and from 25 to 30 per cent. in *Raja batis*. The places where these occur are numerous: in the body cavity, upon the splanchnic (gut) mesoblast, on the subintestinal veins, in kidney tubules, in the pericardium, in the liver, in the skin, in any part of the gut epithelium, especially in the rectum. . . Undoubtedly, many of these germ-cells degenerate, and few, if any, of the vagrant ones, after a certain early period, ever find their way to the germinal nidus [ridge].[3(p58)]

As he studied other species of fish and then amphibians, in each case he discovered numerous "vagrant" germ cells scattered in the various somatic tissues of the adult organism. Over time, he came to suspect that theseabnormally positioned cells persisted as a fact of life in all higher animal species, though by the time his book was published, their existence had not yet been confirmed in humans.

As Beard writes:

> So far (1911) they have only been found from fishes to reptiles; but from various considerations it is not open to doubt that they occur even in the highest vertebrates, and in man himself. Apparently they have been noted by Roux and Barfurth in the frog, and by me in the salamander (*S. maculosa*). In all the embryos yet studied by me under a certain age—*i.e.*, within the limits during which germ-cells are easily found in embryos—no single embryo examined has been devoid of them.
>
> The mode of the development and the life-cycle, in practically all its details, are the same in mammals as in fishes, and unquestionably the whole organization and development of man follow closely along, but along higher lines than, those of a fish. It is therefore concluded that, could one but hit upon some easy method of distinguishing germ-cells during the early development of man and mammals, the occurrence of vagrant ones in various parts of the body, skin, pericardium, pylorus, rectum, liver, kidney, etc., would be as common a phenomenon here as in the fishes.[3(p77)]

However, it wouldn't be until long after Beard's death, during the second half of the 20th century, that scientists would rediscover these "vagrant" germ cells, growing far away from the gonads in various somatic tissues of the adult organism, in mammals and in man.[32] Embryologists now take these vagabond germ cells, appearing out of place, for granted.

Though those that survive most often live out their lives quietly, hidden away in some tissue, should one of these vagrant germ cells be coaxed into dividing by some molecular signal still undiscovered, they can form the rare tumor, teratoma, consisting of a mixture of embryonic ectoderm, mesoderm, and endoderm tissues.[32] These neoplasms differ from other forms of cancer because they contain a variety of differentiated tissues growing in a bizarre, disjointed manner, such as skin, teeth, hair, and cartilage thrown together almost randomly. These strange growths prove that germ cells possess the genetic capability, if stimulated, to form all the major adult tissue types under certain circumstances, even after lying dormant for years. No other cell type in the adult organism can do this. In a sense, germ cells have a certain totipotency, like the cells of the blastocyst during early embryonic development.

Though pathologists in the late 19th century had identified teratomas, Beard first made the claim that these tumors grew from a misplaced germ cell, as has now been confirmed.[4(p2)] But Beard believed his vagrant germ cells might explain far more than an occasional teratoma, and indeed would help link together his ideas about the trophoblast and cancer of all forms and types.[3(p87)]

One hundred years ago, scientists vigorously debated the origins of cancer, as they continue to debate the issue today. We are amazed, in reading through the scientific literature of Beard's time, how little seems to have changed over the decades. By 1900, researchers in Europe had proposed a number of theories to explain the formation of malignant cells, with each school of thought vigorously defended. Though they might argue over the fine points, most scientists in the cancer field accepted as fact that the disease develops in the process referred to as "metaplasia," or "metaplasy," in which mature, well-mannered, highly differentiated somatic cells in our tissues and organs mutate into primitive, poorly differentiated, aggressive, invasive tumors.[3(p67)]

For most of the past century, the majority of academics accepted this process as fact, though no one really knew with any certainty how a mature normal cell might so transform. A 1964 publication of the old United States Department of Health, Education, and Welfare entitled *Science and Cancer* presented the official dogma of the day, largely unchanged from Beard's time, that cancer forms in a stepwise fashion from normal mature healthy cells:

> We must again emphasize that although for the convenience of discussion we refer to cancer, there is no sharp all-or-none difference between normal cells and cancer, but rather a series of transformation from the temporary, benign hyperplastic

masses, to benign tumors that remain localized and non invasive, through dependent neoplasms that can continue to grow and invade only if certain hormonal or other conditions of the host are met, to cancers with varying degrees of normal appearance and normal functions, to the relatively completely independent anaplastic cancer without any recognizable normal functions ...

We have also referred many times to "the cancer cell." . . . The stimuli that convert normal cells to cancer cells are not limited to an individual cell, but must affect a population of cells, and it is more than probable that similar changes then take place in many cells of the cellular population.[33(pp90-91)]

As neatly packaged as this explanation may appear, no scientific evidence ever backed up the hypothesis (above stated as fact) that cancer, usually if not always, originates from normal tissue that first turns into a benign tumor before transforming into less aggressive, then more aggressive malignancy.

As Beard turned his attention more and more to cancer, by 1900 he had come to reject the generally accepted hypothesis of his day that malignant tumors arose from normal well-differentiated somatic cells. Such thinking seemed to Beard, never one to be patient with his opponents, preposterous, lacking proof, and devoid of common sense:

Under "metaplasy" pathologists understand change in the character of tissue-cells, even in later life . . . Regarding "metaplasy," as little as a man can return to his childhood, so little can any of the cells of his body take on embryonic characters, or change their nature. If any one small part of the body can do this, why not grant the same superhuman power to the whole?[3(p67)]

Beard instead proposed that cancer must originate from one of his vagrant germ cells prodded into dividing, but in a manner and form quite different from the proliferation that creates a teratoma. As Beard writes, speaking of germ cells:

If they do not degenerate, and degeneration is probably often their fate, they may come to lie somewhere or other in the embryo, even in its sexual organs . . . Probably it may be regarded as sufficient if there be in every development at least one, three, or seven such, which, if they do not degenerate, may become the seed of later tumours.[3(p93)]

How would a germ cell give rise to a malignant cancer? According to Beard's hypothesis, a vagrant germ cell, in any location, once dividing, could follow one of two possible pathways. If it tries to give rise to an embryo directly, it forms a teratoma, the bizarre tumor well documented even in Beard's day. Beard fervently believed that such neoplasms represented misplaced attempts of a totipotential germ cell to create an embryo, with all three tissue types represented but without first proceeding through gametogenesis—the usual first step.

In contrast, the vagrant germ cell might try and create gametes, in accordance with its more typical biologic destiny. In this case, Beard claimed, a misplaced gamete, produced in this way in some extragonadal tissue, would in turn give rise not to a teratoma, but instead to an invasive trophoblast, growing in the wrong place at the wrong time, which then becomes cancer. By 1902, Beard came to believe that all cancers, other than the special case of teratoma, occurred when the totipotential vagrant germ cell, hidden away in some organ, formed gametes and from these, the trophoblast. As he writes:

Most, if not all, true tumours are pathological manifestations of some portion of a life-cycle, and they are due to abnormal attempts at development on the part of aberrant germ-cells, derivatives of the cleavage . . . [3(p78)]

With enormous confidence, he states:

In 1902 the conclusion was reached that cancer was (an) . . . irresponsible trophoblast, and in these words for the first time in human history the nature of cancer was laid bare.[3(p131)]

Beard fully realized his proposal presented certain difficulties that needed to be resolved. During normal embryonic development, he had insisted that the trophoblast developed from the fertilized egg before the inner cell mass first appeared. Beard certainly made a strong case for this sequence of events, as we have seen, a chronology now proven by contemporary research. But this usual process of trophoblast formation required just that, a *fertilized egg*. In his cancer hypothesis, Beard claimed that vagrant germ cells gave rise to an aberrant gamete, from which grew the trophoblast, both in women and in men, without the step of fertilization.

For his hypothesis to hold true, as a start Beard needed to explain how a vagrant germ cell in a male sitting in some tissue somewhere might create a trophoblast which normally requires the presence of an egg, and a fertilized one at that. The germ cells of females indeed give rise to eggs, but those in males only produce sperm. So while it's plausible that a vagrant germ cell in a female might yield an aberrant egg, and then an aberrant trophoblast, the scenario seems unlikely in males.

Beard really didn't have a firm solution to this problem, but simply assumed that in both males and females, the vagrant gamete, whether egg or sperm, when prodded into activity in its abnormal location could generate the trophoblast. As Beard writes:

> But why should a vagrant germ-cell, when developing into a cancer, omit or skip the formation of an embryo, and proceed with a different portion of the life-cycle? . . . one is inclined to suppose that it is not immediately due to the further development of a vagrant germ-cell itself: that this latter first of all divides many times, as it would do if in the germinal nidus, and that it ultimately forms more or less normal forerunners of gametes, öocytes or spermatocytes. These would be in abnormal situations and under abnormal conditions, and, under some stimulus, they would develop as though parthenogenetically, but abnormally, to form a trophoblast.[3(pp60-61)]

Beard was more correct in his reasoning than he could ever have realized, though the evidence to help support his thesis wouldn't appear for some 90 years. We now know that in humans, vagrant germ cells, when they do become active *often form oogonia*, the precursors to the female egg, *in both adult men and women*. Carlson, who apparently knows nothing of Beard or his writings, makes this point when discussing the migratory patterns of germ cells during embryogenesis:

> Some primordial germ cells follow inappropriate migratory pathways, leading them to settle into extragonadal sites. These cells normally start to develop as oogonia [the precursor to eggs], regardless of genotype [sex]; they then degenerate. In rare instances, however, they persist in ectopic sites, such as the mediastinum [the chest] . . . [4(p377)]

If these vagrant germ cells can produce eggs in both sexes, then Beard's hypothesis of the aberrant trophoblast becomes somewhat more feasible. But even with this solution now provided, another problem remains, how this *unfertilized egg* might yield a trophoblast, which normally develops only after fertilization.

In the paragraph from his book quoted earlier, Beard referred to parthenogenesis, which provided to him additional evidence that a vagrant germ cell, or its offspring gametes, could start replicating spontaneously without the need for fertilization. Parthenogenesis, first described in the 18th century, refers to the process in which an unfertilized egg develops into a full-fledged organism. In Beard's day, biologists had documented the phenomenon in many arthropods such as aphids as well as in social insects such as the honeybee and the ant. In these species, eggs, if unfertilized, give rise to the male drones, but if fertilized, yield the female workers and queens.[34]

Though rare in vertebrates, under the right conditions parthenogenesis does occur, even in mammals, though the process usually ends in an incompletely developed or otherwise abnormal offspring. However, in 1900, the scientist Charles Loeb successfully produced a fully functional frog by pricking an unfertilized frog egg with a needle. In 1936, long after Beard's death, Gregory Pincus stimulated parthenogenesis in an unfertilized rabbit egg by manipulating its chemical environment.[34]

So in the process of parthenogenesis, an unfertilized egg—the direct offspring of a germ cell—will start dividing and can begin the developmental process. To Beard, it seemed eminently possible that a vagrant germ cell sitting amidst some somatic tissue could do the same. Should the active germ cell take the direct path toward embryonic development, a teratoma results. If instead the germ cell first divides into gametes, then the irresponsible trophoblast might follow, with fertilization unnecessary in either case.

Beard faced other obstacles to make his thesis more scientifically sound. In 1900 scientists accepted—and today many scientists still believe—that cancer arises from mature, differentiated somatic cells gone awry, we suppose primarily because malignant cells tend to resemble, under the microscope, those from the tissue of their origin.[16(pp142-150)] In appearance, cells of a primary brain cancer resemble somewhat normal neurons, leukemia cells look to a certain degree like normal white blood cells, a pancreatic cancer cell, as invasive and deadly as it can be, mimics the cells of the healthy pancreas. Of course, the similarities are not exact, and the more aggressive the cancer, the less it approximates in appearance the tissue of origin. But even in very aggressive cancers, pathologists can see similarities between the tumor cells and cells of the normal tissues in which they grow. It seemed reasonable 100 years ago and seems reasonable today to many to assume that cancer must arise from mature differentiated cells.

To Beard, the physical similarity of cancer to differentiated somatic tissues said nothing about their origins, nor was he surprised that his aberrant trophoblasts might resemble the tissue in which they grew. He suspected that the local environment of the germ cell affected the actual histological appearance of its offspring trophoblast. As Beard writes:

> In this way it [the germ cell] becomes an irresponsible trophoblast, and it may imitate or mimic anything in its environment. Whatever it mimics—something existent or non-existent—it is always an "imitation tissue," and behind the domino or mask an irresponsible trophoblast.[3(p134)]

As so often was the case, Beard was way ahead of his time. Twenty-first century embryologists and contemporary molecular biologists have confirmed that the environment of a cell profoundly influences its development, including its appearance. Earlier, we mentioned that in the mammalian blastocyst, if the inner cells of the morula are moved to the surface, they transform into trophoblasts, and if trophoblasts on the outside are transplanted to the inside, they soon look and behave like early embryonic cells.[4;12] During the development of the pancreas gland, undifferentiated precursor cells, if exposed to connective tissue, or mesenchyme, form enzyme synthesizing, exocrine cells. If they fail to contact the mesenchyme, these same precursors give rise to the endocrine, hormone-secreting pancreatic islets.[4(p339)] Such events, the rule in developmental biology, illustrate that the molecular environment of a cell helps determine its ultimate destiny, the type of cell it will become. So in light of 21st century science, Beard's proposal really isn't all that implausible; it seems almost predictable that if a vagrant germ cell did begin proliferating, its trophoblastic offspring would adopt the appearance, at least to some degree, of the host tissue.

The germ cell origin of cancer does help explain another phenomenon widely documented in Beard's day, and extensively studied today, the abnormal chromosomes found in many, if not all cancers. The nuclear chromosomes contain our DNA, the basic genetic machinery of the body and, in cellular terms, appear fairly large in size, large enough to be seen in the light microscopes of the 19th century. By the early 20th century, scientists understood that every species studied had a fixed number of matched, paired chromosomes: humans, we now know, have in all somatic and germ cells 23 pairs, or 46 total chromosomes. On the other hand, the chromosomes in cancer cells frequently appear under the microscope abnormal, in terms of both number and their appearance.[16(p154)] In malignant cells, chromosomes often form duplicate sets, or incomplete sets with some apparently randomly deleted. At times, sections of individual chromosomes seem to be missing, or translocated to another chromosome where they don't belong. Most experts in the field today consider such aberrations, such chromosomal mutations the essence of cancer itself, so rarely will any malignant cell have the expected complement of normal chromosomes.

Dr. Michelle M. Le Beau, writing in *Cancer: Principles & Practice of Oncology*, in one sentence sums up current thinking about cancer and chromosomes, writing: "The malignant cells in virtually all patients who have leukemia, lymphoma, or a solid tumor have acquired chromosomal abnormalities . . . "[35(p103)]

In his writings, Beard alluded to such chromosomal aberrations, very much aware that cancers differed from normal somatic tissues in this regard. However, he did not accept the consensus of his colleagues, that these abnormalities represented the *cause* of cancer, instead offering a very different explanation for their appearance.

Beard believed cancer grew as an aberrant trophoblast originating from a vagrant germ cell. In the more normal course of events in adults, germ cells give rise to gametes through meiosis, in which a single germ cell with a full complement of chromosomes—23 pairs, or 46 total chromosomes in humans—ultimately divides into four gametes, each with 23 total chromosomes, half that found in the somatic cell line. In this process, the chromosomes of a germ cell first duplicate, producing two sets in the cell for a total of 92 chromosomes. The germ cell then undergoes two divisions, ultimately resulting in four gamete offspring each with 23 chromosomes. When two gametes, an egg and a sperm, combine in fertilization, each brings with it half a set of chromosomes so that the union results in a full, paired collection.[4(pp3-8)]

In Beard's model, the vagrant germ cell tries to recreate the life cycle of the organism, out of place and at the wrong time. Since germ cells are the direct precursors of gametes, this misguided cell replication might include efforts at meiosis with duplications and divisions of chromosomes. Since all of this would be happening outside the proper environment of the gonads, this aberrant cell activity, he believed, might easily give rise to abnormal complements of chromosomes, as commonly observed in most cancers. To Beard, the bizarre chromosomes seen in cancer cells seemed not unusual but predictable, reflecting the thwarted attempts of the vagrant germ cell to form gametes in a misplaced effort at meiosis, a throwback to its normal biologic responsibility.

We would again like to quote Dr. Beard's own words, in discussing his thoughts about chromosome abnormalities and cancer. In the following, he uses the term mitoses instead of meiosis but the thought is the same:

> In view of all this, the events in a malignant tumour—such as, for example, the "heterotype" [abnormal] mitoses—lose much of their importance. They may still possess an interest for the cytologist and embryologist, and even a passing one for the pathologist. But to the physician and surgeon these abortive attempts to form gametes cease in treatment to have any import whatsoever.[3(p120)]

But other nagging questions remain. Why would a vagabond germ cell, sitting in some tissue or organ, remain quiescent for years or even decades, then suddenly spring to life and try to begin a new life cycle? What could make the germ cell behave so inappropriately in the first place? Beard, writing from the perspective of his time, tried to address this issue:

> Such a persistent embryonic germ-cell, encapsulated within the individual, may at any time, by illness, injury, irritation or other cause—such as declining years—weakening the system, be awakened into activity.[3(p134)]

Such a statement might seem simplistic by modern standards, but in one sense Beard does address the process of inflammation, one of the most active areas in contemporary cancer research. Scientists today who may know nothing of Beard and his trophoblastic-germ cell theory of cancer, do believe that an excessive inflammatory response to cellular injury, coupled with cellular damage due to aging or exposure to toxic free radicals, can induce the formation of malignancy.[12;36]

But once stimulated into action, why does a vagrant germ cell decide occasionally to form an embryonic teratoma, and more commonly a trophoblastic cancer? What determines the specific direction a germ cell will take? Beard did not have precise answers for this question, and admitted as much. But since these misplaced germ cells were located far removed from their preferred home of the gonads, he suspected they would be subjected to a multitude of local influences and signals, depending on the host tissue, that could affect their developmental path. Given the limitations of the science of his day, it isn't surprising Beard could not be more specific. The steroid hormones, so essential for embryonic and trophoblastic survival as well as for gametogenesis, wouldn't be identified until the 1920s. And scientists wouldn't really appreciate the importance of growth factors, crucial during the process of implantation, until the 1990s. Perhaps these molecules might influence the vagrant germ cell, helping to determine how it behaves and what it becomes.

# CHAPTER 5

# Germ Cells and Stem Cells: Proof for Dr. Beard?

**C**an we point to any contemporary evidence that might help link Beard's mutant trophoblast, growing from a wayward germ cell nestled away in some tissue somewhere, directly to cancer? We believe such documentation does exist, documentation that propels Beard's thoughts about "vagrant" germ cells and the "trophoblast as cancer" right into the middle of one of the most active research areas in molecular biology today—the origins, behavior, and therapeutic application of stem cells. Hardly a week passes without some major media venue reporting the latest advance in the field, the next great hope for stem cell therapy, and the latest political debate about the ethics of using embryonic stem cells for medical purposes. Arguments pro and con about the potential of stem cells and their practical application in medicine have reached right into the White House, eliciting more than one Presidential pronouncement.

To help bring Beard into the 21st century, and into the modern world of stem cell biology, we need to return back to the early embryo. Previously, we mentioned that two days after conception, at the four-cell stage, each cell if isolated has the potential to form a complete normal embryo. By day three, the embryo consists of some 12–16 cells, but by this point each individual cell has lost some of its development potential. None by itself can grow an entire embryo, but each can still give rise to any tissue or organ.

Early in the third week after conception, the inner cell mass separates into the upper epiblast, the future embryo body, and the lower hypoblast, from which the yolk sac eventually forms. As these two cell lines diverge along their unique developmental paths, by the end of the third week the epiblast itself begins separating into three tissues that serve as the foundation for all future body structures: an upper segment of cells, the ectoderm; a middle segment, the mesoderm; and a lower segment, the endoderm, resembling a three-layered cake (See Figure 12). The ectoderm eventually matures into the skin and the nervous system tissues, including the eye and auditory apparatus in the ear. The mesoderm ultimately forms all bone as well as the cartilage that lines joints, the other connective tissues, the muscles including the heart, and the vessels of the circulatory system, both arterial and venous. The endoderm gives rise to the lungs and the entire digestive tract with the associated organs, including the stomach, intestines, liver, gallbladder, and pancreas.[4(pp59-74)]

As the embryo evolves from the amorphous early epiblast into ectoderm, mesoderm and endoderm, researchers believe that the individual cells become still more limited in terms of their developmental capabilities. Cells of the early ectoderm can only form ectoderm structures, such as nerves or skin, not muscles or the lining of the intestinal tract. Cells of

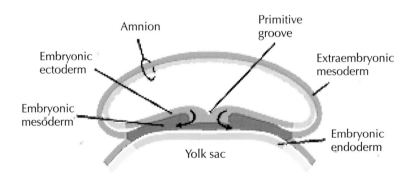

**FIGURE 12:** The three primitive tissue layers: ectoderm, mesoderm and endoderm.

*(Originally published in Carlson BM: Human Embryology & Developmental Biology, 4th Ed., St. Louis, Mosby, 2008. Copyright Mosby 2008. Used with permission.)*

the early mesoderm can give rise to connective tissue and its relatives such as muscle, but never neurons or intestine. And cells of the endoderm can mature into the extraordinarily complex tissues of the digestive system, but cannot, most believe, become nerve or muscle cells.

At each step during embryonic growth—from the fertilized egg, to the morula, to the blastocyst, to the epiblast with its three essential layers—the capacity of the individual cells to create different tissues and organs becomes more and more restricted.[37] Each of the first four cells after fertilization can form an entire embryo; the cells of the morula and early blastocyst can grow into any cell type but not an entire embryo; the cells of the ectoderm, mesoderm and endoderm have even less developmental flexibility.[38] And finally, the mature differentiated cells of each of our tissues, such as the neurons of the brain, the connective tissue and muscle cells, the cells of the intestinal tract and pancreas, have no ability under normal conditions to be anything other than what they are, be it a nerve, a muscle, an intestinal mucosal cell or pancreatic epithelium. In fact they cannot even produce duplicates of themselves, for these mature, differentiated cells *do not ever themselves divide, for all practical purposes.*[27(p510)]

As a fundamental rule of molecular biology, in a complex organism, as cells become differentiated they lose their ability to replicate. In contrast, single cell organisms, such as a paramecium or bacterium, can divide endlessly, allowing for the survival of the species; in a sense, such humble creatures have an immortality not found in the differentiated cells of complex tissues of multicellular organisms.

In "higher" animals such as ourselves, in the mature organism only certain cell lines retain the capacity to divide: the germ cells of the ovaries and testes, the source of the gametes; fibroblasts, the class of cells that synthesize connective tissue and the ground substance of organs; and stem cells—the final link between Dr. Beard's thesis of 100 years ago and contemporary molecular biology.

Currently scientists recognize two types of stem cells, embryonic and adult. The embryonic variety consists of the blastomeres of the early blastocyst, those primitive undifferentiated cells that replicate rapidly and mature gradually into the complex tissues of the trophoblast and the fully formed, fully differentiated fetus. By definition, each embryonic stem cell retains the ability to grow an entire organism from scratch. In contrast, the adult variety includes those stem cells located in all the tissues of our various organs where they remain for the duration of our lives. These cells, when stimulated into action, can divide, creating mature differentiated versions of the tissues in which they reside.

For the official government definition of stem cells, we would like to excerpt the statement from the National Institutes of Health website:

### What Is a Stem Cell?

A stem cell is a cell that has the ability to divide (self replicate) for indefinite periods—often throughout the life of the organism. Under the right conditions, or given the right signals, stem cells can give rise (differentiate) to the many different cell types that make up the organism. That is, stem cells have the potential to develop into mature cells that have characteristic shapes and specialized functions, such as heart cells, skin cells, or nerve cells.[38]

We personally find the Wikipedia discussion far more comprehensive:

**Stem cellular structures** are cells found in most multicellular organisms. They are capable of retaining the ability to reinvigorate themselves through mitotic cell division and can differentiate into a diverse range of specialized cell types. Research in the stem cell field grew out of findings by Canadian scientists Ernest A. McCulloch and James E. Till in the 1960s. The two broad types of mammalian stems cells are: **embryonic stem cells** that are found in blastocycts, and **adult stem cells** that are found in adult tissues. In a developing embryo, stem cells can differentiate into all of the specialized embryonic tissues. In adult organisms, stem cells and progenitor cells act as a repair system for the body, replenishing specialized cells, but also maintain the normal turnover of regenerative organs, such as blood, skin, or intestinal tissues.[39]

The best technical definition of adult stem cells we've located appears in an article by Stanley Miller and colleagues:

> Organs are composed of collections of differentiated cells that perform discrete functions. An underlying homeostatic system exists to replace senescent differentiated cells and tissue loss following injury. This hierarchical system typically involves several stages of cells that have decreasing reproductive capacity and simultaneous increasing commitment to differentiation. The most primordial cell in the hierarchy, the *stem cell,* has the ability to reproduce for the life of the organ. It is typically undifferentiated, divides infrequently, and often resides in a specialized physical locale termed a "niche." Following division, a stem cell will give rise to, in average, one daughter stem cell that will remain in the stem cell niche and another, variously termed a *transit-amplifying cell* in most epithelial studies . . . These rapidly proliferating cells undergo further reproductive divisions . . . . and progressively commit irreversibly to differentiation along one or several lineages.[31]

In summary, stem cells, both embryonic and adult, have certain defining characteristics: histologically, they appear primitive, undifferentiated under the microscope.[31] In terms of their location, embryonic stem cells are by definition only found in the earliest blastocyst stage, whereas adult stem cells have been identified in every one of our 200 distinctive tissue types.[38] In terms of their behavior, both embryonic and adult stem cells possess unlimited replicative potential, coupled with the ability to form mature differentiated tissues.

Thirty years ago, when researchers first began their investigations, they believed that adult stem cells inhabited only certain tissues, such as the bone marrow or along the lining of the intestinal tract where rapid cell turnover occurs. To early students in the field, their appearance in these two sites seemed eminently logical; after all the cells of the intestinal mucosal lining slough off approximately every five days, requiring rapid regrowth. Stem cells nestled in the intestinal crypts allowed for this rapid regeneration, continuing for the many decades of the normal human lifespan. Since red blood cells live on average about 120 days, our entire supply must be replaced every four months—a prodigious feat, again made possible by the stem cells in the bone marrow, the site of all blood cell production.

Outside of the intestinal crypts and bone marrow, in other tissues with only an occasional need for new cells, researchers initially believed that the old differentiated cells could somehow start dividing to generate the needed replacements. In some locations, such as the brain and muscles, in which cells can live for the lifespan of the organisms, it was thought these cells, should they die, could never be replaced. We now know that stem cells inhabit even these two sites, and with proper signaling, they can reproduce to replace damaged neurons or muscle cells.[38]

Theoretically, both embryonic and adult stem cells can proliferate end-lessly, but under normal circumstances their rate of replication varies enormously from tissue site to tissue site; the small intestinal mucosa must regenerate every five days, the red cells of the blood, every four months, but neurons can last a lifetime.[40] So, though any stem cell from any organ potentially can divide indefinitely, the process must be tightly controlled locally by very precise molecular signaling, to avoid cellular excess or deficiency within a particular tissue.[31]

Adult stem cells can actually replicate along one of two pathways, as Miller et al above imply; they can reproduce, but remain undifferenti-ated to maintain the supply of stem cells, or, depending on prevailing signals, they can mature into the various differentiated tissues of a com-plicated organism.[31] In this regard, they serve as a reservoir of cells available as needed to replace those lost due to normal turnover (as in the intestinal lining), injury, disease, or aging.

If the stem cell offspring mature along a differentiated route, they invari-ably lose this ability to divide. Drs. Robert G. Fenton and Dan L. Longo, in their excellent review of cancer cell biology in *Harrison's Principles of Internal Medicine,* sum up nicely current concepts about differentiation, stem cells, and cellular replication:

> In tissues with rapid turnover, such as skin, bone marrow, and gut, an individual cell is on one of two largely mutually exclu-

sive paths: division or differentiation. Cells capable of dividing are undifferentiated (stem cells), whereas terminally differentiated cells are unable to divide. Stem cells produce daughter cells that can either become new stem cells (thus replenishing the stem cell compartment) or undergo terminal differentiation, depending on the circumstances and the environmental signals.[27(p510)]

As one of the more perplexing mysteries of modern molecular biology, scientists have absolutely no idea where or how these mysterious adult stem cells originate, despite the millions of dollars of research investment over the past 40 years. We know of course about the origins and developmental route of embryonic stem cells, which arise from the fertilized egg in pathways known since Dr. Beard's day. But no one knows how and where adult stem cells first appear. Some believe that they must be holdovers from embryonic growth, but however logical it might seem on first glance, this thesis remains unproven.

For the official NIH position on the subject of stem cell origins, we would like once again to excerpt a quote from their site:

> Unlike embryonic stem cells, which are defined by their origin (the inner cell mass of the blastocyst), adult stem cells share no such definitive means of characterization. **In fact, no one knows the origin of adult stem cells in any mature tissue** [bold ours]. Some have proposed that stem cells are some-how set aside during fetal development and restrained from differentiating.[41]

Within years of their discovery, researchers began to contemplate the therapeutic possibilities of stem cells. Scientists were impressed that these cells seemed capable of renewing tissues quite effectively, and at times, as in the intestinal mucosa or bone marrow, quite rapidly. If this replicative potential could be harnessed and appropriately directed, theoretically stem cells might be used to repair tissue affected by disease or injury, or even replace entire organs, such as a heart catastrophically damaged by myocardial infarction.

The NIH website rather enthusiastically portrays the possibilities of stem cell therapies:

> Another potential application of stem cells is making cells and tissues for medical therapies. Today, donated organs and tissues are often used to replace those that are diseased or destroyed. Unfortunately, the number of people needing a transplant far exceeds the number of organs available for transplantation. Pluripotent stem cells offer the possibility of a renewable source of replacement cells and tissues to treat a myriad of diseases, conditions, and disabilities including Parkinson's and Alzheimer's diseases, spinal cord injury, stroke, burns, heart disease, diabetes, osteoarthritis and rheumatoid arthritis.[42]

Despite the optimism, after many years of research, the only practical application has been the use of marrow stem cells in bone marrow transplant therapy, itself of limited value.

Bone marrow transplantation, or more correctly in its current incarnation, stem cell transplantation, has proven most effective against diseases of the marrow cell lines, such as inherited immunodeficiency diseases, leukemia and lymphoma.[43] In the procedure, patients undergo high dose chemotherapy, often along with total body radiation, to obliterate the diseased bone marrow. Subsequently, hematopoietic (marrow) stem cells from a genetically compatible donor are infused intravenously into the patient. These "foreign" stem cells, by a very precise homing mechanism, eventually make their way to the marrow where they restore the depleted cell lines. Theoretically, the process offers great promise, but the obstacles have been many. As a start, most studies report that at least 10% of patients undergoing the procedure die as a consequence of the treatment, with mortality rates described as high as 30–50% in cases of an unrelated but matched donor.[43-45] Then, the transplant can fail for any number of reasons, or the newly formed immune cells with the donor's genetic identity can start attacking the tissues of the host patient in the potentially deadly graft-versus-host disease. Even if the transplant does take hold without significant damage to the host, in cases of leukemia and lymphoma nests of cancerous cells can survive the induction therapy, allowing the disease to recur.[43]

Adult stem cells have been employed to treat Parkinson's disease, diabetes, even advanced kidney cancer, with inconclusive results. And the dream of regenerating entire organs remains just that, a dream.[42]

Research in the field has provoked considerable controversy in recent years, in part because of the perceived limited developmental capabilities of the adult stem cell line. Scientists have long believed that these cells derived from some mature organ site can only replicate cells of that tissue, and no other type. That is, bone marrow stem cells can only produce red or white cells, not liver cells or intestinal mucosal epithelium. Liver stem cells can only differentiate into hepatocytes, not red blood cells or intestinal mucosa epithelium. This limited replicative repertoire differs considerably from the unlimited potential of the earliest embryonic blastomeres, each of which can form an entire body with all its complex tissues.[31]

In 1998, Dr. James Thomson and his group at the University of Wisconsin isolated human embryonic stem cells, which they then successfully grew in culture, providing scientists with the hope of unlimited supplies of totipotential cells to replace entire organs.[42] Debates about the ethics of harvesting such human embryonic stem cells continue to rage, with no let-up in sight. Some scientists recently have proposed that adult stem cells may possess far more "plasticity" than was previously believed, that is, they may have the ability to form multiple differentiated tissues, not only the type from which they were extracted.[38] For example, recent studies show that in both mice and humans, transfused bone marrow stem cells will, in the liver, form hepatocytes, not red or white blood cells.[46;47] If such findings prove true, adult stem cells, properly manipulated, might serve as efficiently as the embryonic variety to provide a source of healthy replacement tissues without all the controversy.

So, how does modern stem cell research in any way relate to Dr. Beard, his theories of vagrant germ cells, and the trophoblast as cancer? Of course, Beard never used the term "stem cell," a phrase that wouldn't enter the scientific jargon until the 1960s. But he did talk about germ cells, the precursors of the gonadal ova and spermatogonia, a cell line we would once again like to consider in this context.

Beard correctly described the maturation of these perplexing cells outside of the embryo in the yolk sac of the hypoblast. He also helped map out the journey of these cells back to the primitive hindgut of the embryonic body, then along a predetermined and circuitous path within the embryo itself, ultimately terminating in the gonads. He also reported that during this rather extraordinary journey, many germ cells follow a divergent course away from the gonads, ending up in the various developing tissues in all the organs in the embryo, where they remain alive for the duration of the host's adult lifetime.

Beard had also identified his "vagrant germ cells" as the origins of teratoma, that peculiar tumor consisting of a variety of differentiated tissues mixed together in a near random fashion. From his studies of this odd neoplasm, Beard knew his vagrant germ cells could begin dividing to create all three basic embryonic cell lines, the ectoderm, mesoderm, and endoderm, from which under normal circumstances all our tissues and organs ultimately develop.[3]

My pathology text from medical school, Robbins' *Pathologic Basis of Disease*, provides the modern interpretation of this tumor, which confirms Beard's claims from 80 years earlier:

> These tumors are derived from totipotential cells having the capacity to differentiate into elements representative of any of the three germ layers—ectoderm, mesoderm, and endoderm . . .
>
> Mature solid teratomas are comprised of a heterogeneous, helter-skelter collection of differentiated cells or organoid structures such as neural tissue, muscle bundles, islands of cartilage, clusters of squamous epithelium, structures reminiscent of thyroid gland, bronchial or bronchiolar epithelium, and bits of intestinal wall or brain substance, all embedded in a fibrous or myxoid stroma.[16(p1226)]

Many of Beard's other findings about germ cells have stood the test of time, to become accepted scientific dictum. For example, he understood that germ cells appear under the microscope as primitive and undifferentiated in structure. He knew too that these cells had enormous capacity for division, as evident in their normal activities within the ovaries of females and testicles of males. In females, ovarian germ cells begin replicating during late embryonic life, giving rise to the precursor eggs which continue to mature over a period of many years. The germ cells can continue dividing throughout the decades of active fertility, right up until menopause, when the follicles atrophy and their activity comes to a close. In men, the process follows a somewhat different route; testicular germ cells do not begin proliferating until puberty, when spermatogenesis first begins, but thereafter, they continue replicating, at least to some extent, for the duration of the host's lifetime.[4(p2)]

So if we sum up some 20 years of Beard's research, he described and defined his vagrant germ cells as histologically primitive and undifferentiated, dispersed in all the tissues of the body, with the potential to divide at any time during the lifetime of the host, and with the ability to create all the various differentiated tissues of the body. As we review Beard's descriptions and definitions of these cells, we could think of no better description or definition of what we today call adult stem cells, those primitive, undifferentiated cells dispersed in all the tissues of the adult body, with the potential to divide at any time during the lifetime of the host, and with the ability to create all the various differentiated tissues of the body.[31] In some respects, germ cells are by definition the ultimate stem cell, in the gonads giving rise to the gametes (eggs and sperm) that when merged create a single cell capable of forming a complete, functional adult body. But all that growth and development starts with the germ cells.

Recent evidence does help make the case that Beard's vagrant germ cells are identical to stem cells. In a 2006 paper, Turnpenny and colleagues reported that early embryonic germ cells do possess the same totipotentiality as do embryonic stem cells:

> In mammalian biology, two clear sources of untransformed pluripotent stem cell have been described. The inner cell mass (ICM) of the early embryo gives rise to the derivatives of all three germ layers in the developing embryo. Taking the ICM into in vitro culture offers the opportunity to derive embryonic

stem cells (ESCs). These cells, first attained from mouse embryos by Evans and Kaufman and, independently, by Martin in 1981, retain the ability for broad differentiation but also undergo self-renewal. As such, they are the pluripotent stem cell that has been the focus of most research. An alternative source of pluripotent cells arises later in development. Germ cells are the sole means of transmitting genetic information to the next generation in their ultimate form as haploid gametes, spermatozoa, and ova. However, before meiosis, these cells exist as diploid primordial germ cells (PGCs). PGCs share significant similarities to the cells of the ICM and, once taken into in vitro culture, can lead to the generation of embryonic germ cells (EGCs), the parallel of ESCs.[48]

With all this evidence before us, we believe that 100 years ago, in his exacting analysis of vagrant germ cells, their microscopic appearance, geography, and behavior, Dr. Beard identified adult stem cells, though of course he never used that modern term. We also believe that he long ago solved a mystery that still perplexes students of the field to this day, the origins of adult stem cells. If Beard's vagrant germ cells are indeed adult stem cells, his discovery that they mature in the yolk sac far removed from the embryo body provides the long sought answer to this particular riddle.

We do believe Beard deserves long overdue credit for discovering stem cells, and describing much of their behavior as well as their origins, but he didn't have the complete picture. Though in his writings he comes close, he never quite says that these vagrant germ cells he described actually serve a useful function under normal circumstances, as a reservoir of cells in all our mature tissues, providing a near endless supply of replacements for those lost due to normal turnover, injury, disease, or aging. But he seems to have gotten just about everything else right, in terms of the basic biology of the adult stem cell line.

In Beard's writing, his impressive discoveries about germ cells took secondary place to his main concern—or perhaps obsession—the origins of cancer. Though he trained as an embryologist and biologist, not as a physician or medical researcher, his doctoral thesis covering a most esoteric of subjects, the development of the sense organs in a small parasitic worm, all his investigations from the earliest seemed to pull him toward cancer, its origins, and ultimately, its treatment.[49]

By 1905, with the trophoblastic origins of cancer decoded, Beard began arguing his case in the medical journals, at conferences, and later in his 1911 book, that cancer arose directly from an aberrant trophoblast, growing from a vagabond germ cell stimulated into frenetic reproductive activity.[3] In Beard's day, most cancer researchers in the Western world insisted otherwise, claiming that cancer arose only from mature differentiated cells located in a mature differentiated tissue, that through some unknown process transformed into an undifferentiated phenotype, then began wildly dividing without restraint, and through a series of unknown steps acquired the ability to invade, migrate through tissues, and create new blood vessels—in a way no other normal tissue, other than the trophoblast, was known to do. But despite Beard's impressive evidence, his opponents stuck to their guns, always trying to debate and argue and attack him into appropriate scientific submission. To them, his ideas about vagrant germ cells, parthenogenesis, and wayward trophoblast as cancer seemed ludicrous, if not simply insane.

When I (Dr. Gonzalez) was in medical school at Cornell in New York in the early 1980s, during our second year pathology course eminent scientists from the medical school itself, and from our sister institutions Rockefeller University and Sloan-Kettering, lectured us about malignant disease, particularly its origins. The prevailing thesis, at least in the lectures, had changed little in the 80 years since the debate raged over Beard's trophoblastic hypothesis. We were taught that cancers, all cancers, arose from the mature differentiated cells in the various tissues of our body that through some bizarre unknown process turned into primitive, undifferentiated beasts with a whole new set of abilities, the capacity to invade, to migrate, and to create new blood vessels needed to sustain the growing tumor. Though no one could explain how such a series of implausible events might happen, how a mature healthy differentiated cell might so completely transform, the experts that taught us all knew that cancer happened just this way. Of course, my professors pointed to the usual suspects to explain this phenomenon—genetic aberrations, the favorite culprit, wrought by defective inheritance, or through acquired mutation in the DNA, the result of bad luck, or provoked by carcinogenic environmental exposures, etc. etc. etc., but still, no one seemed able to explain this extraordinary process of cellular metamorphosis.

Despite what the lecturers might have said, during my medical school years the tide had already begun to shift somewhat. Though I remember our teachers sticking to the ancient canons about the formation of cancer from differentiated normal cells, the textbooks already hinted at something else. In my pathology class at Cornell, we used the 1979 Second Edition of the classic text, *Pathologic Basis of Disease* by Drs. Robbins and Cotran, which I still turn to nearly 30 years later, and which I earlier referenced. In the chapter entitled "Neoplasia" the authors discuss the evolving thesis about the origins of malignant cells, which we excerpt below. Note that here the authors now use the word "anaplasia" in place of the older word "metaplasy," to refer to the concept that adult differentiated cells give rise to cancer:

> Little is known about the cellular origins of benign neoplasms; they may arise from adult-type differentiated cells. *Cancers, on the other hand, are thought to arise from reserve or stem cells* found in all specialized tissues. Thus, an undifferentiated cancer results from proliferation without differentiation of reserve cells. Similarly, the well-differentiated cancer probably also arises from primitive reserve cells that undergo specialization as they proliferate to create the neoplasm. The conceptual issue is more than academic. While many specialized cells lose their capacity to replicate as they become fully mature (e.g., the upper layers of stratified squamous epithelium), in neoplasia specialization may occur without loss of replicative capability.
>
> Anaplasia may be used as a synonym for undifferentiation of tumor cells. Literally, anaplasia implies dedifferentiation, **a phenomenon that is now no longer believed to occur** [Bold ours]. Nonetheless, the term anaplasia has come to have specific connotations with regard to neoplasms. *Anaplastic tumors are invariably malignant and are composed of more or less un-*

*differentiated cells that have lost some or all resemblance to their normal counterparts.*[16(pp146-147)]

Despite the prescient comments of Drs. Robbins and Cotran, another 20 years would pass before such concepts became widely accepted within the research community, whose members for most of that time still held to the cherished belief that cancer formed from differentiated normal cells. Even as recently as the 15th Edition of *Harrison's Principles of Internal Medicine* published in 2001, the authors of the chapter "Cell Biology of Cancer" report that the disease developed from a single differentiated cell undergoing mutations "caused by intrinsic errors in DNA replication or are induced by carcinogen exposure."[27(p510)]

The situation began to change rather dramatically when in 1997 Bonnet and Dick at the University of Toronto first reported the origins of acute myeloid leukemia, not from mature differentiated neutrophils, but from hematopoietic stem cells, whose normally tightly regulated proliferative behavior had gone awry.[50-52]

Then in 2003 a group at the University of Michigan announced their startling findings that the culprit in breast cancer may not be mature differentiated cells but breast stem cells, again proliferating without their characteristic restraint.[53]

A press release from the University dated February 24, 2003, stated the breast cancer case:

> ANN ARBOR, MI—Of all the neoplastic cells in human breast cancers, only a small minority—perhaps as few as one in 100—appear to be capable of forming new malignant tumors, according to just-published research by scientists in the University of Michigan Comprehensive Cancer Center. The discovery could help researchers zero in on the most dangerous cancer cells to develop new, more effective treatments.
>
> "These tumor-inducing cells have many of the properties of stem cells," says Michael Clarke, M.D., a U-M professor of internal medicine, who directed the study. "They make copies of

themselves—a process called self-renewal—and produce all the other kinds of cells in the original tumor."

Although similar cells have been identified in human leukemia, these are the first to be found in solid tumors, Clarke adds. The cells were isolated from primary or metastatic breast cancers removed from nine women treated for cancer at the U-M's Cancer Center.

The discovery—reported this week in the online early edition of the Proceedings of the National Academy of Sciences—also may explain why current treatments for metastatic breast cancer often fail, says Max S. Wicha, M.D., an oncologist and director of the U-M Comprehensive Cancer Center.

"The goal of all our existing therapies has been to kill as many cells within the tumor as possible," Wicha says. "This study suggests that the current model may not be getting us anywhere, because we have been targeting the wrong cells with the wrong treatments. Instead, we need to develop drugs targeted at the tumor's stem cells. If we are to have any real cures in advanced breast cancer, it will be absolutely necessary to eliminate these cells."[54]

The researchers at Michigan isolated these stem cells from breast tumors, then injected them into mice, all of whom in turn developed the malignancy. To the surprise of the investigators, a small number of these stem cells could generate a substantial and aggressive cancer:

"As few as 100 to 200 of these tumor-inducing cells, isolated from eight of nine tumors in the study, easily formed tumors in mice, while tens of thousands of the other cancer cells from the original tumor failed to do so," Clarke says . . .

. . . Given that tumor-inducing cells now have been identified in breast and blood cancers, Wicha and Clarke believe it is likely that similar cells drive the development of other types of cancer as well. The U-M Comprehensive Cancer Center is establishing a new research program to identify stem cells in other cancers and develop new therapies to destroy them.

"What we are working on now is finding out what makes these tumor stem cells different from the other cells in a tumor," Wicha says. "Now that we can actually identify them, we can start developing treatments to specifically target and hopefully eliminate them."[54]

Two years after Wicha's original report, in 2005 Dirks at the Hospital for Sick Children, Toronto, linked aberrant stem cells to brain cancer.[55;56] Then in February 2006, the American Association of Cancer Research convened a workshop to bring together the experts who now believe cancers of numerous types originate from the stem cell line.[57] That year Wicha et al published a long article entitled "Cancer Stem Cells; An Old Idea—A Paradigm Shift," summarizing the accumulating data to that time linking stem cells to a variety of cancers.[58] Since then, Wicha's group at Michigan has identified stem cells as the culprit in pancreatic cancer, and Friel et al at Massachusetts General Hospital reported their discovery of stem cells as the "tumor initiating cell" in endometrial malignancy.[59;60]

In an interview published in the May 5, 2006 issue of *Oncology News International*, Dr. Wicha described the growing belief among researchers that many if not all cancers, whatever the type or form, might originate from stem cells. We thought the article significant enough to excerpt pertinent paragraphs below:

## Growing Evidence Supports Stem Cell Hypothesis of Cancer

BETHESDA, Maryland—During the past 18 months, researchers have developed substantial evidence supporting the notion that stem cells play a critical role in the development of at least some cancers, their progression, and the prognosis of patients, including breast, brain, lung, and prostate cancer, multiple myeloma, and melanoma.

"The idea of stem cells in cancer is a very old one, but it is only recently that scientists have had experimental models that actually validate this," Max Wicha, MD, professor of internal medicine and director of the University of Michigan Comprehensive Cancer Center, Ann Arbor, said at a meeting of the National Cancer Advisory Board (NCAB). "It represents a paradigm shift in how we need to approach cancer, because it has very wide clinical implications."

The stem cell hypothesis challenges the classic stochastic model, which holds that cancer results from a random mutation in a cell that reproduces and eventually forms a malignant neoplasm. In contrast, the stem cell model suggests that in many instances, stem cells or their immediate progeny are the cells transformed during carcinogenesis, and that only these cells are capable of self-replication within a tumor. All other cells in a cancer have lost their ability to self-renew and are in various stages of differentiation.

Moreover, if these differentiated cells should escape the primary tumor and travel to other parts of the body, they would not grow metastases of clinical consequence. This means that once a cancer develops, its growth is driven by a small number of cells—perhaps as few as 100—which have the two distinguishing properties of stem cells, namely the ability to make exact copies of themselves and to differentiate . . .

"If the stem cell model is correct, then we have to reexamine, in a very critical way, the preclinical models for therapeutic development," Dr. Wicha said. "We have to look at the endpoints for clinical trials, which may not be adequate because the tumor stem cells may be resistant to these therapies. And we think effective therapies will need to target the tumor stem cells population . . . "[61]

After discussing the Michigan group's latest efforts, the author reports:

The stem cell model, if confirmed, carries enormous implications for oncology. In Dr. Wicha's view, identifying and eliminating mutated stem cells, or forcing them to differentiate, may one day become an important prevention strategy . . . .

Thus, effective therapy and, perhaps, prevention would need to focus on the stem cell underlying a cancer. Killing a tumor's differentiated cells but not its driving stem cells may explain why patients have tumor shrinkage that has no impact on their survival. "We need to be targeting the stem cell population," Dr. Wicha said.[61]

If for a moment we allow that Dr. Beard's vagrant germ cells were indeed what we today call stem cells—and we believe undoubtedly they are—then the elegant research and insightful proposals of scientists like Dr. Wicha have really helped bring his trophoblastic thesis on the origins of cancer full circle, or at least nearly so. Dr. Wicha's model still lacks one essential component—the trophoblast. He and his colleagues believe cancer forms as a stem cell begins replicating uncontrollably, without any intermediary steps. Remember, Dr. Beard insisted that malignant disease did not develop directly from a vagrant germ (stem) cell sitting in some tissue, but rather from its trophoblastic product—formed when the process of gametogenesis begins in response to some aberrant signal, in the wrong place and at the wrong time. The resulting gamete, presumably an egg, then moves along its own parthenogenic embryonic journey, next giving rise to the aberrant trophoblast, fully able to invade, migrate, create vessels, and metastasize easily to distant organs.

If, with the work of Dr. Wicha et al, we now can link cancer with some comfort to stem cells, and if we are willing to identify stem cells with Beard's vagrant germ cells, does any contemporary evidence exist that might in turn associate cancer directly with aberrant trophoblast, the final missing link in the Beardian hypothesis on the origin of cancer?

Earlier, we discussed the molecular mechanisms, the four transcription factors Hxt, Oct-4, Mash-2, and Hand-1 that help determine whether a trophoblast, during its early development, remains undifferentiated and invasive, or matures into the syncytiotrophoblast bereft of any aggressive demeanor.[8;20] Recall that Hxt-4 appears at the earliest stages of embryogenesis, instructing a number of uncommitted primitive blastocysts to form rapidly dividing, invasive trophoblast.[18] During this same period, Oct-4, a differentiation factor, remains suppressed.[22;23] Later, the nuclear levels of Mash-2, which further drives trophoblastic replication and aggression, begin rising while those of Hand-1, responsible for a more indolent phenotype, stay low.

In the nucleus of the trophoblast, Hxt and Mash-2 activate cyclin and cyclin-dependent kinase systems, which signal DNA to start replicating, and in turn, the cells to continue dividing. In contrast, Oct-4 and Hand-1, which when present guide the formation of the syncytiotrophoblast, inhibit these same signaling cascades.[19]

We know that the same processes and the same exact helix-loop-helix proteins are at work in the cancer cell. In malignancy, the cell nuclei express high levels of Hxt and Mash-2, each of which activates the cyclin system and DNA replication, followed by rapid cell division. All the while, the concentration of the differentiation factors Oct-4 and Hand-1 remain quite minimal, repressed, as in the early trophoblast.

During the early stages of trophoblast life, the cyclin B levels are three times higher than when the cells become less invasive at eight weeks of gestation.[8;25] In cancer, cyclin B activity similarly stays elevated, permitting the cells to replicate and invade.[35(p123)]

We have also seen that as the trophoblast transforms into a collection of quiescent giant cells, the tumor suppressor gene p21 turns on in response to rising levels of Hand-1. Subsequently, p21 directs the synthesis of an enzyme that shuts down the entire cyclin/cdkB proliferative signaling system.[25] In cancer, Hand-1 remains repressed as does the p21 tumor suppressor gene, further freeing cell proliferation from any molecular restraint. With Hand-1 absent and p21 dormant, the malignant cell line can continue dividing, invading, and migrating without inhibition.

Finally, in both the trophoblast and cancer, with Hxt and Mash-1 active, with the cyclin/cdkB proliferative signaling system fully operational, with replication unhindered, the cells become essentially immortal, immune to the usual cellular fate (in complex organisms) of apoptosis. When Oct-4 and Hand-1 predominate—as happens in the less aggressive syncytiotrophoblast and in all non-replicating differentiated tissues—apoptosis becomes the inevitable end.[2;8]

Although the mechanisms of the trophoblast and cancer are endlessly complex, in ways beyond the scope of this discussion, in essence both cell lines seem to employ the identical messenger molecules, identical signaling mechanisms, and identical biochemical pathways, right to the level of DNA transcription. But still other evidence exists linking the trophoblast directly to the cancer phenotype, evidence provided by recent investigations of the hormone hCG.

The early embryo cannot successfully invade the uterus without a steady source of progesterone, needed to keep the endometrial lining receptive. During implantation, the trophoblast itself begins secreting hCG, human chorionic gonadotropin, which ultimately circulates in the maternal blood and stimulates the active ovarian follicle to continue releasing the much-needed progesterone.[6] hCG is therefore a trophoblastic hormone, long thought to be synthesized in no other normal tissue.

Scientists have known for years that choriocarcinoma, the cancer of an uncontrolled trophoblast, and tumors that arise from germ cells such as certain testicular and ovarian malignancies, all manufacture and secrete hCG which can be used as a marker to track the success of treatment. Falling blood levels of hCG indicate possible therapeutic success, rising levels correlate with worsening disease.[17]

Until recently, researchers believed only these rare malignancies, choriocarcinoma and germ cell tumors, synthesized hCG.[27(p494)] With more sophisticated techniques available to measure the protein, we now know, thanks to the elegant work of Drs. H.F. Acevedo and A. Krichevsky and their team, that virtually every cancer studied secretes hCG.[62;63] In a series of rigorous experiments, Dr. Acevedo and his colleagues searched for hCG in 74 different human cancer cell lines and in each case, isolated the hormone.[64] Some cancer types expressed more of the hormone than others, but they all produced it. As Dr. Acevedo et al report:

> The expression of the membrane-associated epitopes [types] of hCG and its subunits was found to be a phenotypic marker characteristic of all evaluated cultured human cancer cell lines, irrespective of their type or origin. There were, however, quantitative and qualitative differences in the expression of the different epitopes.[64]

Would there be any advantage for a cancer cell to secrete hCG? If we think about the normal trophoblast, its successful invasion of the uterus requires signaling between it and the local endometrial epithelium, and close cooperation between these two tissues. Progesterone promotes such synergy, without which implantation fails. In a parallel manner, a malignancy, wherever it first appears, may release hCG locally in a calculated attempt to help make the nearby environment more receptive to invasion.

Such evidence from contemporary molecular biology seems to bring us closer still to Dr. Beard, and his hypothesis that cancer not only looks and behaves *like* trophoblast, but that cancer *is* trophoblast, always and only. We believe that the evidence points nowhere else.

# Conclusion to Part I

When we think about Dr. Beard, we can but marvel at his extraordinary achievements, particularly given the time in which he worked, and the relatively primitive tools available to him. Yet, through pure hard work and rather remarkable intelligence, he successfully unraveled many mysteries of embryonic growth and development in vertebrate animals, including humans. We believe unquestionably that in his vagrant germ cells he identified what we now call stem cells, some 60 years before they would be rediscovered by McCulloch and Till. Without the accoutrements of the modern laboratory, he proved, we believe conclusively, that cancer did not develop in some magical process from mature, differentiated tissues, but only from germ-stem cells via their gamete offspring and the trophoblast, in mammals the only truly invasive tissue—other than cancer—ever identified.

When Beard died in 1924, his trophoblastic thesis had already been relegated to the footnotes of arcane medical history. True, some of his less controversial discoveries, such as the journey of the germ cells from the hypoblast, have become accepted scientific canon. But his major achievements—his discovery of stem cells, and his claim that cancer may very well arise from misplaced trophoblast—remain to this day unappreciated, ignored by the overwhelming majority of mainstream cancer researchers, all of whom we believe could learn so much from a journey into the Englishman's world.

# PART II

# The History of the Enzyme Treatment of Cancer

# Introduction to Part II

As we have now seen, Dr. Beard was the first to report that in many respects the trophoblast in its early form looks and behaves like a typical malignant tumor. It begins growing as a very undifferentiated offshoot from the primitive blastocyst, its cells proliferating almost without control, as tumors were known to do even in Beard's day. The trophoblast then adeptly invades the mother's uterus, much as a cancer infiltrates host tissue in any organ,[1;2] and it quite efficiently produces a dense blood supply—a requirement for any rapidly growing neoplasm, as angiogenesis research today has made very clear.

As normal development proceeds, however, at some predetermined point the trophoblast transforms from this undifferentiated, rapidly dividing, highly invasive, angiogenic tumor-like tissue, into the non-proliferating non-aggressive mature placenta. Beard realized in this remarkable metamorphosis, trophoblast differs fundamentally from malignancy, which unless effectively treated never stops replicating and never stops invading.

During the early years of Beard's career, he became obsessed with this change in trophoblast appearance and behavior that ultimately distinguishes this tissue of pregnancy from malignancy. For he believed if he could unravel the key, the cause of this transformation, if he could understand why the trophoblast, so like a tumor initially, changed so drastically, he might have the solution to cancer.

In an earlier chapter, we discussed the works of insightful researchers such as Ferretti and her group from Italy, and Murray and Lessey from North Carolina, who have meticulously catalogued the molecular and biochemical similarities between the early invasive trophoblast and malignancy.[1;2] Certainly, both groups have in great elegant detail demonstrated the similarity between the two tissues. However, neither addresses the phenomenon familiar to all students of embryology, that as aggressive and as cancer-like as the early trophoblast may be, at some point—usually about 8 weeks after conception in humans—it routinely undergoes its remarkable change. One would suppose that researchers in the field, aware as they are today of the similarity between the two tissues, would be intrigued, as Beard came to be, that the trophoblast drastically alters its developmental course while cancer does not. But this rather extraordinary difference between the two, its hows and whys, Ferretti et al and Murray and Lessey do not, except in passing, discuss.

Beard spent more than a decade of his life seeking an answer to this riddle, trying to learn what ultimately determined the fate of the trophoblast, eventually concluding that the key to its metamorphosis resided in the embryonic pancreas. As witnessed in every species of mammal he studied, the day the embryonic pancreas becomes initially active, synthesizing and secreting its coterie of enzymes, the trophoblast ceases its cancer-like invasion of the mother and begins its evolution into the mature, non-aggressive placenta.

Even in Beard's day, more than 100 years ago, the main categories of pancreatic enzymes had already been identified: the proteolytic, or protein digesting component; the lipases that hydrolyze triglycerides; and the amylases, responsible for cleaving complex carbohydrates into simple, easily usable sugars.[65] Physiologists of the time thought all three groups were active only in the duodenum, where the enzymes continue the breakdown of food arriving from the stomach. But Beard, based on his years of study, concluded that above and beyond this function, trypsin, the main proteolytic enzyme, served to control placental growth and prevent the tissue from invading beyond the uterus as a true cancer might.

After reporting that fetal pancreatic enzymes ultimately restrain the trophoblast, Beard then took his investigations—and claims—a major step further. He proposed in a series of lectures and papers beginning in 1902 that since the early trophoblast behaves much as a tumor does, since under the microscope its cells even look like undifferentiated, primitive neoplastic cells, and since the pancreatic secretions forcefully regulate its growth and character, these very same enzymes could be, in fact must be, the body's main defense against cancer, and would be useful as a cancer *treatment.*[66;67]

In 1905 Beard moved from the theoretical to the practical, testing the efficacy of trypsin in the widely used Jensen's mouse tumor model available at the time. In a brief summary appearing in the January 20, 1906 issue of the *British Medical Journal*, he reported his preliminary results, indicating that the injectable enzymes could impressively attack cancer.[68] Though in this first effort Beard treated only two animals, in both cases the tumors ceased their growth and turned necrotic. In the control animals receiving no therapy, the tumors continued to flourish, spreading as per usual.

Shortly thereafter, physicians aware of Dr. Beard's thesis began treating their own cancer patients with injectable preparations of pancreatic enzymes with some significant reported success. In the first case we've been able to track down in the literature, in 1906 a New York physician, Clarence C. Rice, M.D., wrote of a successful response in a patient with cancer of the larynx. [69] In his report, Dr. Rice describes the rapid sloughing of a "tumor covering almost the entire left vocal cord," with the enzyme therapy:

> It seems to me that you will agree with me that this is a remarkable cure. That the growth was removed by the effect of the trypsin injections, and by the pancreatic capsules called "holadin," there can be no doubt, because no other treatment was used.[69]

Unfortunately, the tumor had not been biopsied, so critics questioned the validity of the case. But over the next three years, a number of reports appeared in the conventional medical literature, including *The Journal of the American Medical Association*[70] and *The British Medical Journal,*[71] describing successfully treated patients whose tumors had been appropriately confirmed by biopsy.

We have read as many of these documents as we have been able to track down, and they remain to us compelling evidence of patients surviving advanced cancer—such as one with a fungating sarcoma of the jaw, well beyond any chance of surgical cure, whose tumor under enzyme therapy regressed, then fell off.[3] The patient thereafter resumed a normal, cancer-free life. Other articles describe patients with metastatic colorectal[72] and uterine cancer,[73] as deadly today as in Beard's time, whose disease apparently resolved as a result of the enzyme treatment—all carefully substantiated and appropriately presented in the scientific literature.

The enzyme thesis, and the supporting animal and human data, provoked an enormous and angry backlash against Beard and his followers. He was vilified in medical journal editorials, mocked in the newspapers, belittled at scientific conventions.[74] But he also had strong supporters: in the May 1906 issue of *McClure's Magazine*, a very popular lay publication at the time, a British physician-writer, C.W. Saleeby, published a lengthy defense of Dr. Beard entitled "Cancer-Can It Be Cured?"[75] Dr. Saleeby followed up with a book, *The Conquest of Cancer*,[76] which the New York Times favorably reviewed on January 4, 1908.[77]

Beard himself fought back in articles and letters to the editor, and in 1911, he published *The Enzyme Treatment of Cancer*,[3] the monograph outlining his decades of research and his promising and compelling results. Despite such efforts, interest in Beard's thesis gradually petered out, and when he died in 1924, he died frustrated, angry and ignored, his therapy already considered by most no more than an historical oddity. But through a combination of chance and good luck, others over the years would periodically rediscover Beard's intriguing trophoblastic hypothesis, his impressive laboratory and clinical findings, and fight their own often bitter battles to keep the therapy alive.

# CHAPTER 6

# From Fish to Trophoblast

**B**eard linked the synthesis of fetal pancreatic enzymes to trophoblast destiny through hard labor over a 15-year period that began with his study of a seemingly unrelated subject, the formation of sense organs in a small invertebrate parasite. To understand his rather unusual journey, we need to review, for a moment, the scientific world into which Dr. Beard matured.

At the end of the 19th century, many fine researchers had unraveled the mysteries of early development in complex organisms, both plant and animal. In the field of botany, scientists had made sense out of the complicated life cycle of plants, which included an alternation of generations, that is, a sexual generation alternating with an asexually reproducing form.

In all higher plants, the asexual organism is dominant—the large plant we all know well, such as a tulip, a rosebush, or a 200-foot redwood tree. This asexual form gives rise within the flower to spores that in turn develop into the very inconspicuous sexual generation, both male and female, replete with their own sex organs. Usually, the sexual offspring appear as miniscule structures within the flower, incapable of living on their own. In this environment, they release their gametes, which then come together to form a zygote, the plant embryo, which as it matures creates a seed, the end result of the sexual union. Should the seed find its way to fertile soil, upon germinating it grows into another dominant asexual plant, rooted to the ground, and the cycle starts anew. Botanists knew in Beard's day that the asexual generation in plants, including trees, has the theoretical potential for unlimited growth, until restricted by available nutrient supply.

By 1900, biologists had uncovered this complicated life cycle not only in plants, but in certain "lower" animals as well, such as the jellyfish. In these invertebrates, in contrast to plants, the *sexual form* dominated, while the asexual generation appeared small in stature, undistinguished and decidedly unimpressive. For example, in true jellyfish, technically called Cnidarians, the well-known large globular floating organisms with their tentacles represent the sexual generation with its two genders, each with highly developed sex organs. Male and female of the group respectively release sperm and eggs into the surrounding seawater. After fertilization, the eggs then develop into small, free swimming larvae that eventually attach to rocks or the ocean floor itself. Once rooted, these larvae mature into polyp-like forms, the *asexual* generation, which release large numbers of spores into the surrounding water. These then hatch into minute free-swimming medusae that eventually mature into the sexual generation of the common jellyfish, both male and female. In this complicated life cycle, the sexual and asexual forms are each completely independent organisms, one a predatory jellyfish, the other a miniscule polyp firmly rooted to the seabed.

In more complex animals such as humans, scientists assumed no such alternation of generations existed. The life cycle of vertebrates including the mammals, so it was thought, involved only a sexual generation, with its two distinctive genders, but never an intervening asexual form. Each mature sexual organism produces gametes, either eggs or sperm depending on its sex, that when combined during fertilization yield a single-celled zygote. This then develops directly, the teaching goes, into a new sexual being. In Beard's day scientists universally accepted this linear pattern in vertebrates as they do today, that proceeds simply from gametes to zygote to adult to gametes to zygote. Not only did zoologists discount the existence of an asexual generation in vertebrates, they argued that this streamlined, direct development helps differentiate us from the lowly plants and lower animals.

By the time Beard finished his Ph.D. studies at the University of Freiburg in 1884, he considered the direct formation of the sexual embryo from

the fertilized egg in vertebrates, without an intervening asexual generation, an important, fundamental biological law. As he writes:

> Like my fellow-workers, I had been taught to regard the develop-
> ment of any of the higher animals as "direct"; that is to say, from
> the fertilized egg a new sexual organism, a worm or a fish, a bird or
> a man, arose directly. From the tissues or soma of this sexual or-
> ganism new reproductive products, eggs or sperms, sprang. In this
> way the simple cycle of "egg-sexual organism, egg-sexual organ-
> ism" repeated itself *ad infinitum*.[3(p144)]

During his stint as a graduate student at Freiburg, Beard concentrated
his efforts on the embryology of invertebrates, with their complex alternation of sexual and asexual generations. His Ph.D. thesis detailed the
specific life cycle of the genus myzostoma, a small parasitic worm with a
complicated life, that lived on and off of still larger worms.

During the mid-1880s, Beard left invertebrates behind, to focus his attention on the morphogenesis of the nervous tissue in fish. In 1885, he
published a lengthy monograph, "The System of Branchial Sense Organs and Their Associated Ganglia in Ichthyopsida."[78] Then in 1889, he
completed a comprehensive report summarizing his study of the sense
organs, including the eye, of various fish species. During this period,
Beard appeared to have been quite productive, on the secure road of
carving out a niche for himself in this very specialized area of biology,
except for an odd turn of events. In 1888, while associated with the
Anatomical Institute of the University of Freiburg, he received a grant to
study at a biological research center located on Black Lake in the
Adirondacks of New York State. During his summer in that New World
wilderness, Beard chose to study the freshwater billfish, a diminutive
cousin of the rather spectacular group of long-jawed sport fishes that includes the well known salt water marlins, sailfishes and swordfishes.
These legendary game fishes provided considerable sport for Ernest
Hemingway during his Cuba days. Our casual Internet search for
"Billfish" pulled up 51,000 references, many devoted to their conservation, more it seemed dedicated to their role as game fish.

Beard spent his time in New York unraveling the embryology of the billfish nervous system, from its earliest appearance. Like most fish, billfish

begin their lives ensconced within a small egg floating around unattached in the surrounding lake water, with its yolk providing nutrition. In his usual meticulous style, Beard made hundreds of microscope slides chronicling the step by step sprouting of nerves in the diminutive billfish embryo. Once back in Germany, as Beard began studying these specimens, to his surprise he observed a phenomenon never before reported for any vertebrate species.

Scientists had already discovered by the 1880s that in the fertilized fish egg, the earliest structure that appears is the blastoderm, thought to be separate from the future fish body, an extraembryonic structure equivalent to the yolk sac in mammals. Though this small tissue had been accurately described, no one prior to Beard had any idea what function it might serve. But in his examination of his own specimens Beard detected something that seemed at first preposterous, a primitive nervous system within the blastoderm growing completely independently of any embryonic body tissue, evident before any of the fetal tissues could be observed. This set of nerve cells persisted for a time before degenerating and disappearing completely; furthermore, the blastoderm withered only after the embryo itself began forming with its own set of nerves, the forerunners of the nervous system of the adult fish. These findings left Beard somewhat perplexed because it seemed that during development in this organism, he had observed two separate, very distinctive collections of neurons, one appearing before any sign of the embryo and separate from it, the other, as part of the fetus itself. The embryo's nervous system, which did not appear to originate from the blastoderm, could be observed only as the blastoderm vanished.

Subsequently, Beard identified the same unusual sequence of events in other species of fish he studied, as well as in the completely unrelated amphibians. None of this made any sense at all to him, given what he had been taught about the embryology of vertebrates. During their very linear development only a single nervous system should be evident, growing inside the embryo where it belonged—not two sets, one forming only after the other disappeared. Beard himself thought his findings implausible until he began to consider the complex life cycles of plants and the "lower" invertebrates such as jellyfish. He suspected, initially somewhat cautiously, that in these "higher" animals, i.e. the billfish and salamander, he had witnessed an alternation of generations, the cycling over time of an asexual form, the blastoderm, with the sexual organism, a phenomena that all experts categorically knew did not, could not, and should not happen in any vertebrate species. But the primitive nervous system of the blastoderm he had seen over and over again, that first group of nerves destined eventually to disappear, must be, Beard reasoned, the nervous system of the asexual generation that predates the dominant sexual embryo with its own sophisticated collection of neurons.

If indeed he was correct, if he was witnessing an alternation of generations in fish, it made sense to Beard that the asexual generation would be insignificant, almost vestigial, then degenerate before the embryo itself began to flourish. In the lower animals such as the jellyfish, in which an alternation of generations had already been definitively identified, the asexual organism always appeared diminutive and undistinguished. So Beard thought it reasonable that the higher one looked in the animal kingdom, the more complex and dominant would be the sexual form, the less impressive would be the asexual. That's why, Beard proposed, the asexual generation in vertebrates had never been reported—small and fleeting, it had simply escaped observation.

Beard knew his proposal, this alternation of generations in vertebrates, contradicted the accepted dogma, and if proven true, could change profoundly our understanding of the animal kingdom. In his book, he writes of the first inklings that he might be on to something significant:

> My embryological faith was perfectly orthodox when, on June 14, 1888, I left the shores of Black Lake, New York, with an extensive assortment of preserved material of fish development. One of the earliest finds made after the return to the Anatomical Institute of the University of Freiburg in Breisgau was of the existence of two distinct and separate nervous systems in the life history of the bill-fish. . . . About a year later the like find of a twofold nervous apparatus was made in some other fishes and amphibians, and especially in the smooth skate. . . .The transient nervous apparatus of ganglion cells and nerve fibres in the skate development functioned for a time, for about

three months from the start out [of] the total of *circa* seventeen, and then quite suddenly began to fade away, and to undergo a slow but sure degeneration.

The two nervous systems crop up again and again in my published writings since 1888. . . . All my original work, from 1888 down to to-day, is impregnated with facts concerning the two nervous systems, and the antithesis underlying them. . . .[3(pp144-5)]

If the life cycle of fish and salamanders included such an alternation of generations, Beard suspected that the same phenomenon must apply to all vertebrates, even humans. He assumed, in fact predicted, that the asexual generation in higher animals might be small in size, might be transient—like the blastoderm—and might be totally unimpressive, but it must exist in all vertebrate species no matter how lofty, just as it existed throughout the plant kingdom. But Beard had uncovered evidence of an asexual generation in only a few species of fish and salamanders. It was quite a leap of faith to generalize these preliminary findings to all animals, including humans. To make the point convincingly, he still had to identify the asexual generation in mammals, and in man. And it was this search for this elusive organism in humans that would lead Beard to study the mammalian trophoblast.

The term trophoblast, from the root "troph" meaning nurturing, had first been used by A.W. Hubrecht in 1889, just as Beard's own research was gearing up.[3(p125)] Hubrecht and his colleagues reported that in the morula stage of the blastocyst, the cells on the periphery form early trophoblasts, while simultaneously the inner blastomeres give rise to the inner cell mass that eventually develops into the body proper. The trophoblast then gradually matures into the placenta, the anchor and nutritive source for the growing embryo. Since that time, for more than 100 years now, most embryologists have accepted the same chronology claimed by Hubrecht, the synchronous formation of the trophoblast and inner cell mass.

Beard pointed out that this claimed chronology, the alleged appearance of the trophoblast and inner cell mass at the same time, had never actually been *observed*. It was an assumption that had made its way into all the biology texts of the era, and remains in all the texts today. And when Beard studied his many slides of the early mammalian blastocyst, he saw something completely different.

Beard spent thousands of hours viewing specimens of a variety of species including human, donated by women who had spontaneously miscarried. And as a result of his own careful studies, he arrived at a conclusion that put him at odds with his scientific colleagues, suspecting that after fertilization of the egg, *the trophoblast formed first*, before the inner cell mass, in fact before any embryonic cell lines of any kind could be identified.

Beard writes:

> According to orthodox embryology this chorion or trophoblast is a part of the embryo, although it is invariably present before any part of an embryo; although it may persist after the complete disappearance of the embryo; although it is never formed from or by an embryo; and although ultimately it never makes any part of the embryonic body! Logically, how can it be maintained that a structure which arises before an embryo, and out of no part of it, and which never goes to form any part of any organ of the body, is embryonic or fœtal in nature?[3(p90)]

Researchers today, as we have seen, have confirmed Beard's theory that the trophoblast appears before the inner cell mass. But Beard then went yet a step further in his thinking. He proposed that the trophoblast served not just as a mere appendage for nutrition as was commonly believed, but as nothing less than the asexual generation of mammals, directly equivalent to the blastoderm of the billfish or the asexual form of a plant, appearing before the sexual embryo, and giving rise to it.

Beard writes, in summarizing his conclusions:

> Were an embryologist of to-day asked what in outline was the cycle of development in one of the higher forms—say a fish, chick, or mammal—he would probably be amazed at the question. "The hen lays the egg, the latter gives birth to a new hen," and so . . . the cycle is completed.

> In the higher animals—the Metazoa—what is termed "direct de-
> velopment" does not, and cannot, exist. It has been found that
> the cycle of animal development, even of the highest forms, re-
> sembles very closely that of a fern or flowering-plant. In the line
> from egg to egg there are two generations—an asexual form, and
> one which, as it is the bearer of sexual organs, is spoken of as the
> sexual generation.[3(p54)]

But Beard needed to resolve one more issue to prove an alternation of generations in mammals. In the life cycle of plants, a sexual generation produces gametes, which, coming together as a fertilized egg or zygote, then give rise to the asexual generation. The mature asexual organism in turn releases spores, which develop directly into the sexual embryos, male and female, and so the process begins again. Though he had demonstrated to his satisfaction that the trophoblast represented the asexual generation in mammals, no such spores or anything remotely resembling a spore had ever been reported in the life cycle of any vertebrate species.

After much thought and years of research, Beard proposed a solution. In the late 19th century, scientists including Beard had investigated the origins of the sex cells appearing in ovaries and testicles, and their embryonic precursors, the germ cells. In animals such as mice, germ cells were first seen in the posterior epiblast, from which it was universally assumed they must develop. Since the epiblast eventually matures into the three basic tissue layers, the ectoderm, mesoderm and endoderm, and ultimately, the embryonic body, scientists concluded that germ cells arose directly from somatic cells, or at least from their direct predecessors. Embryology texts since that time have taught that germ cells develop from the posterior area of the epiblast as essentially somatic in their origins, akin to every other body cell type from the neurons of the brain to muscle fibers of the toes.

By the late 1880s, embryologists including Beard, remarkably, had also worked out the complex journey of the germ cells outside of the developing embryo body, from the epiblast to the yolk sac and then back again. We say remarkably, because it is extraordinary, given the tools available in the mid-to-late 19th century, that scientists such as Beard could have identified the complex travels of the germ cells, and that these discoveries would hold up to scrutiny today. However, even though germ cells took this unique trip during development, they were still assumed to be somatic cells, though a rather odd breed, maturing for a time outside the embryonic body.

In fact, the somatic origin of germ cells in vertebrates, along with the development of the embryo of vertebrates directly from the fertilized egg, were part of the biological canon Beard learned and accepted early in his studies. As he writes:

> Under this, still generally accepted, conception of development the germ-cells were somatic in origin, and the gradual building up (epigenesis) of a new sexual organism happened directly, when such an egg had been fertilized. Such, briefly, was the simple embryological creed which my teachers, Milnes Marshall, Huxley, and Carl Semper, taught. During some eight or ten of the early years of my original work this was my embryological faith, if an investigator may have any scientific creed.[3(p144)]

In his studies of fish, Beard made an observation that would lead him to question the dogma about the somatic origins of germ cells. He noted that the germ cells of one species he studied, the skate, could first be identified in the early blastoderm, his proposed asexual generation, outside of the embryo body and before the appearance of any of the body tissues. In every species he studied, Beard found that the germ cells seemed to arise before the embryo itself, as the product of the asexual generation, and not—as was universally believed—from the embryo and its epiblastic, or somatic, line of cells. The germ cells might appear in the epiblast of the early embryo at some later time, but despite what everyone else believed, that was not their site of origin. These all-important cells, Beard eventually came to insist, could not be somatic in nature.

Furthermore, during his meticulous studies, he came to suspect that not only did the germ cells appear before the embryo, but one of them was destined to give rise to the embryo itself. The remaining germ cells would then migrate to the epiblast as it formed, to serve as the precursors of the sex cells. It was that simple—*a single cell from the germ line was the progenitor of the embryo, not the other way around*. And Beard, as he thought about the alternation of generations in fish, concluded that this single primordial germ cell he had discovered, the parent of the future embryo, was equivalent to the spore in plants, a product of the asexual generation, and the parent cell of the sexual organism.

Beard confirmed that the embryo grew from a single germ cell in a number of fish species, then in amphibians, but these were still "lower" animals. However, Beard believed he had uncovered a universal rule that should apply to the most complex of animals, and during the mid-1890s, he turned his attention to mammals, their germ cells, and their origins. Eventually, he discovered that the trophoblast, the proposed asexual generation in this group, indeed gave rise to the first, primordial germ cells before any sign of the embryo. And it was one of these germ cells that grew into the embryo! Here they were, the spores not thought to exist in any vertebrate, evident not only in fish and amphibians, but also in mammals. As in the fish he had studied, only one of these germ cells was so destined, he believed, while the others would eventually appear in the posterior epiblast, before beginning their peculiar migration to the yolk sac, then eventually to the hindgut of the growing embryonic body.

In his book, Beard reminisces at some length about the path his work had taken, as he put together his theory on the alternation of generations, and germ cells as the vertebrate equivalent of spores:

> The tracing of the asexual generation in the backboned animals or vertebrata, from fishes to man, was not without its own special difficulties. These were due rather to expecting too much, and to failing at first to realize that the higher one ascended in the scale of life, the greater became the organization of the sexual form or generation, and the more insignificant the asexual one, until in the highest animals, the mammals and man, the asexual generation became reduced to the almost structureless chorion or trophoblast, as Professor A.W. Hubrecht named it in 1889 . . .

> In 1895 the standpoint had been attained that in every life-cycle of a higher animal, such as man, there were two generations: an

asexual one—the trophoblast, and a sexual one—the metazoan individual or person. The puzzle was not how the first of these arose, for clearly it could be demonstrated any day in the week that it was the direct product of the cleaved or segmented egg . . . Somehow or other there arose gradually upon it the sexual generation . . .

How? Something resembling the spore mother cells of plants was required. . . . It was not until towards the close of 1900, when the first harvest of the germ-cell researches had been reaped, that the problem was cleared up. The germ-cells arose before the embryo, as products of a single cell, the primitive germ-cell, in a direct line from the fertilized egg. They came into being upon the asexual generation or trophoblast. To contain and to nourish these germ-cells for a brief span of time another organism was needed, a sexual one, endowed with sexual organs.

How was the sexual organism obtained? . . . There was only one source from which such a sexual generation could arise: this was by the evolution or unfolding—the self-sacrifice—of one germ-cell for the well-being of the rest, and to contain them. At the epoch of the formation of the primary germ-cells, all were alike in origin and potentialities. All were so many potential individuals of the species.[3(pp125-8)]

Beard's proposal that germ cells did not originate from somatic tissues but from the trophoblast, and that one of these served as the primordial spore giving rise to the sexual organism, went far against the simplistic teachings of his day. But it's fair to ask, does any contemporary research support Beard's essential contention that a single totipotential germ cell predates the embryonic body, and gives rise to it?

Earlier, we discussed the work of Turnpenny and colleagues, who have shown that embryonic germ cells possess the same totipotentiality as embryonic stem cells, that is, both cell types have the capability to form an entire organism.[37;48] Taking this similarity a step further, Zwaka and colleagues at the University of Wisconsin essentially *equate* embryonic germ cells (EG) with embryonic stem cells (ES). Furthermore, Zwaka proposes that ES cells may actually originate *from* embryonic germ cells, and not the other way around, confirming Beard's claim that the germ cell was the parent of all embryonic cells. Indeed, the Wisconsin group also identifies embryonic carcinoma (EC)—a laboratory model used to study malignancy—with both ES and EG cell lines. In an article appearing in 2005 entitled "A germ cell origin of embryonic stem cells?" they catalogue the genetic and functional similarities among the three groups—and suggest that germ cells give rise to the other two lines, serving as the fundamental progenitor "stem" cell. In their "Conclusions" they write:

> We hypothesize that ES, EC and EG cells represent a family of related pluripotent cell lines, whose common properties reflect a common origin from germ cells. Although a more detailed transcriptional analysis could ultimately refute the proposed relationship between ES cells and early germ cells, we hope this idea will at least help to stimulate a healthy re-evaluation of what is actually being studied when ES cells differentiate in vitro.

> What is the relevance of a putative close relationship between ES cells and early germ cells? One prediction of this hypothesis is that at least some of the germ cell-specific genes expressed by ES cells, and not by primitive ectoderm cells, are essential for the long-term maintenance of the pluripotent state.[79]

Once again, in his proposal that a germ cell was the ultimate progenitor cell—and not merely the source of future gametes appearing in the epiblast after the embryo has formed—Dr. Beard presciently pre-empted the findings of modern molecular biologists by 100 years. Unfortunately, in his own day Beard was so far ahead of his time that his ideas about the alternation of generations in vertebrates, the trophoblast as the asexual generation, the totipotentiality of the germ cells, and the development of the embryo from a single germ cell were never taken seriously.

Nonetheless, Beard's suggestions about the trophoblast and germ cells, as peculiar as they might have seemed to fellow scientists in his day, would lead him to the next step in his journey, his proposed solution to the cancer problem.

# CHAPTER 7

# The Trophoblast and the Pancreas

By 1900, Beard had unraveled the developmental path of higher vertebrates in great detail. As a start, he believed he had discovered an alternation of generations in all animals, identifying the trophoblast as the asexual organism specifically in mammals, the parent of all germ cells, one of which served as the progenitor spore of the future embryo. But as the 20th century arrived, Beard remained puzzled by what he had first seen in 1889 in his studies of the billfish, the observation that had started his scientific wanderings in the first place. This was his finding that at a seemingly predetermined time, the blastoderm and its primitive collection of nerves began to deteriorate, after the embryo body appears and begins to mature. In all the hundreds of specimens he studied, this precise chronology seemed to hold true.

As his research expanded to other fishes and other species, including pigs and sheep, and eventually, humans, Beard found the same pattern: an initial flourishing of what he called the asexual generation, be it the blastoderm in fish or the trophoblast in mammals, followed by a deterioration—or in the case of the trophoblast, its containment—just at the time the sexual embryo came into its own. He saw this pattern in every species he studied, without fail.

The underlying cause for this chain of events became for Beard an obsession, one that led him back to the billfish and his earlier studies, in which he had first observed the withering of the blastoderm and its unique collection of nerves. He came to suspect that somehow, in its ear-

liest stages of development, the growing fish embryo itself must somehow directly suppress this asexual organism.

As Beard writes:

> Another important question to be solved some fifteen years ago
> was the how and the when of the suppression of the asexual
> generation. This latter, whether represented by the transient
> nervous apparatus and other structures of a fish, or by the tro-
> phoblast of a mammal, went on flourishing for a certain—and
> not very long—space of time, and then, quite suddenly, all
> growth was stopped, and its degeneration was initiated. In years
> long gone by how often have I not watched these asexual struc-
> tures under the microscope, seen them flourish and blossom,
> and then—*subito*, as the Italians say—begin to fade away, as
> though blighted! . . . This led to one of the many little research
> excursions I have made right up the backboned series to the
> mammals, and to the study of human embryos themselves. A
> whole array of interesting and connected events was soon un-
> earthed, and the putting together of these culminated in the dis-
> covery of the critical period—one of the most momentous finds
> ever made![3(p129)]

By this "critical period" Beard meant the precise time in the embryo's
life when the pancreas gland first begins to synthesize and secrete its
complement of digestive enzymes. During his lengthy study of fish embryos, Beard observed that quite early in development, the acinar cells
of the fetal pancreas seemed to be filled with enzyme-containing vacuoles, known as zymogen granules, sitting in the cytoplasm. In the case
of fish, he supposed the embryo required these "ferments" as he called
them to break down the egg yolk, its sole source of nutrition until it
hatched as a free swimming young fish. But in addition, Beard noticed,
as he studied his slides, that at the precise moment he first detected the
enzymes in the embryonic pancreas, the blastoderm—his proposed
asexual generation—began to regress. As often as he checked his findings, Beard found the same sequence of events—just when the zymogen
granules appeared, the asexual blastoderm began to degenerate. From
these detailed observations, Beard concluded that the digestive enzymes

of the embryonic pancreas must somehow be the key, the reason why the asexual generation, in this case the blastoderm, deteriorated.

These were extraordinary observations to have made, requiring intense observation of minute changes in hundreds of small specimens under the microscopes of the 1890s. But Beard then took his discovery a step further. He assumed the blastoderm represented the asexual generation of the billfish, which the embryonic enzymes in turn effectively suppressed. So it seemed logical to him that in a parallel manner the enzymes secreted by the fetal pancreas should similarly influence the growth of the trophoblast, his proposed asexual generation in mammals.

Beard believed his subsequent research, conducted during 1894 and 1895, confirmed his hypothesis. He was the first scientist to report that the embryonic pancreas in a number of mammalian species began synthesizing digestive enzymes quite early in development, 7–8 weeks in humans he claimed, just at the time the trophoblast changed from a proliferating and invasive tissue into the life sustaining and well-behaved placenta.[3(p118)]

Beard reasoned that if, as he had now shown, the mammalian pancreas becomes active in early embryonic life, its enzymes must have a purpose other than digestion. Unlike the fish embryo, dependent as it is on the egg for nourishment, in any mammal the mother's blood supply provides all the nutrients needed in a perfectly predigested form. The embryo takes nothing in by mouth—other than occasional sips of amniotic fluid—so it hardly requires the enzymes for digestion of food until birth. But since the enzymes appeared so early after conception, Beard believed they must be doing something, and that something had to do with the trophoblast.

In his "Introduction," he makes this point:

> . . . at a certain period of development every normal embryo, or soma, or sexual individual, commenced to suppress the trophoblast or asexual generation of normal development. This came to pass by the initiation of the functioning of the sweetbread or pancreas-gland, with its powerful ferments, the two chief of which are trypsin and amylopsin.[3(p25)]

Later, he makes the point yet again:

> The pancreas functions throughout fœtal life in a mammal,
> though it has nothing to digest except the trophoblast. During
> fœtal life the pancreas gland is pouring out its secretion into an in-
> testine which at the present day contains no food to be digested,
> for the food of the fœtus has been prepared by the pancreatic di-
> gestion of the mother. To the fœtus *in utero* this alkaline digestion
> is of no direct use, but it has an indirect import in acting upon tro-
> phoblast. . . If the secretion be absent, neither the asexual struc-
> tures of a fish development nor the cells of chorio-epithelioma
> [choriocarcinoma] do, or can, degenerate.[3(p118)]

Though he had no direct proof, he assumed the embryonic pancreas secretions must control trophoblast growth in humans as well. As he
writes:

> The critical period in a fish or mammal or man is that at which
> the embryonic organs as a whole first begin to function. . . If a
> certain thing happen [sic] at the critical period of a fish, or a mar-
> supial, I know from experience that something corresponding to
> it will take place at the like period in a higher mammal or a man
> . . . Otherwise there would be no essential unity in the mode of
> the development. Undoubtedly, under the action of the pancreatic
> ferments, the asexual structures of a fish development begin to
> degenerate, and, as represented by the trophoblast, they do the
> like in a mammal or a man.[3(pp134-6)]

Beard built up his complex thesis on the origins of cancer in a step-wise
fashion, over a twenty-year period. By 1895, he had unraveled what he
believed to be an apparent alternation of generations in higher vertebrates, identifying the trophoblast as the asexual generation in mammals, and a primordial germ cell its spore. By 1902, he had brought together his thoughts of malignancy as misplaced and uncontrolled
trophoblast developing from a vagrant germ cell. In 1904 he reported
his findings that embryonic pancreatic enzymes were responsible for the
normal degeneration of the asexual generation in vertebrates, including

the trophoblast in mammals. The following year, in a January 20, 1905 lecture delivered in Liverpool, he first presented his thesis that since pancreatic enzymes such as trypsin ultimately suppress trophoblastic growth in the uterus, and since cancer was trophoblastic in origin, trypsin must represent the body's main defense against cancer and would be useful as a cancer treatment. And the controversy that continues to this day began in earnest.

# CHAPTER 8

# Pancreatic Enzymes During Fetal Life

In his study of fish embryos, Beard discovered that the fetal pancreas began manufacturing enzymes very early on, at the time the extraembryonic blastoderm first began to recede. Eventually he concluded that in like manner the embryonic pancreas of humans becomes active fairly soon after conception, at the end of week 7, just at the time the trophoblast begins transforming from an undifferentiated wildly invasive tissue into the more differentiated, non-aggressive and mature placenta.

In his book, Beard describes in some detail his findings relating to the human fetal pancreas:

> In some of the textbooks of physiology stands the statement that the human pancreas at birth "contains trypsin and the fat-decomposing ferment, but not the diastatic one [amylase]"; but, as I know from my comparative observations of years past, its activities really commence at the time the anus is formed, early in the seventh week of gestation . . . the pancreas functions throughout fœtal life in a mammal, though it has nothing to digest except the trophoblast.[3(p118)]

So one reasonably might ask: Does evidence from contemporary embryology confirm what Beard claimed 100 years ago? First, does the human fetus begin manufacturing pancreatic enzymes very early in its life; and second, does this activity truly coincide with the transformation of the trophoblast into the less aggressive mature placenta?

Documentation in the recent scientific literature does seem to back Beard on both counts. Twenty years ago, Colombo et al of the University of Milan, Italy, studied fetal levels of the three main classes of pancreatic enzymes: the proteases, lipases, and amylases. They reported their findings in a 1989 article entitled "Serum Levels of Immunoreactive Trypsin During Development: Comparison with Levels of Lipase and Amylase."[80] In their investigation, these researchers measured maternal as well as umbilical vein blood levels of the various enzymes in 19 fetuses legally aborted at week 14 for "psychosocial reasons." To their surprise, the fetal samples contained significantly higher levels of trypsin than the maternal blood, but lower levels of amylase and lipase—two enzymes Beard never claimed exerted any significant influence over the trophoblast. So certainly, by week 14, the human embryonic pancreas not only synthesizes and secretes proteolytic enzymes, but in amounts higher than those of a normal healthy adult woman. Beard would have expected as much.

In this study, the Milan group only looked at fetuses aborted at week 14, not earlier, so they can provide no information about enzyme production before that time. Presumably, with blood concentrations higher than those of the mother at 14 weeks, one can assume synthesis of the proteases must begin sometime earlier.

In a 1995 paper, "Expression of Pancreatic Enzymes (α-Amylase, Trypsinogen, and Lipase) During Human Liver Development and Maturation," Terada and Nakanuma of the Kanazawa University School of Medicine, Kanazawa, Japan, evaluated the presence of the three classes of enzymes in the fetal and adult liver and gall bladder tissue, as well as the fetal pancreas.[81] Though we think of these enzymes as solely of pancreatic origin, the authors report their production in the liver and gallbladder in fetuses and at times even in adults. As they write:

> Our recent studies have shown that intrahepatic large bile ducts, septal bile ducts, and peribiliary glands express α-amylase isozymes, trypsinogen, and pancreatic lipase in normal livers and in various hepatobiliary diseases.[81]

In their research, Terada and Nakanuma searched for the enzymes in both pancreatic and non-pancreatic tissues specifically during embryonic development. As part of their study, they evaluated 31 livers from human fetuses obtained from either spontaneous abortion or still birth, ranging in age from 9–40 weeks. They also assessed liver tissue biopsy specimens from five neonates, six infants, 16 children, and eight adults, all with no history of liver disease. For three fetuses aged 12, 13 and 15 weeks of gestation, Terada and Nakanuma also measured enzyme levels in the embryonic pancreas itself. They report:

> The immature acinar cells of the pancreata of the fetuses (12, 13 and 15 weeks' gestation) showed moderate and diffuse cytoplasmic positivity for pancreatic α-amylase, trypsinogen, and lipase . . . The adult pancreatic acinar cells showed strong positivity for all three enzymes . . . [81]

So in the earliest specimen available, that of the 12-week-old fetus, the pancreas synthesized enzymes in not inconsequential amounts, putting the time of significant production at least two weeks before the 14 weeks reported by Colombo. Again, we can assume that they must be present even earlier than 12 weeks. We also find this study definitive since the authors directly evaluated the fetal pancreatic tissue, not umbilical blood, for enzyme levels.

In their article, they also discuss the first appearance of the three pancreatic enzymes in the early fetal liver:

> Immunoreactive pancreatic α-amylase, trypsinogen, and lipase were weakly expressed in the immature hepatocytes from *9 to approximately 25 weeks' gestation* [italics ours]. The expression was relatively stronger in the periportal immature hepatocytes. After approximately 26 weeks' gestation, there was no expression in the hepatocytes.[81]

So, not only does the embryonic pancreas begin synthesizing fairly substantial levels of enzymes by week 12, but trypsin appears in the fetal liver at least by week 9, the earliest specimen available.

Terada and Nakanuma also suggest that the fetal hepatocytes secrete enzymes directly into the embryonic bloodstream, allowing them to circulate systemically. Once in the general circulation they would inevitably make their way into the trophoblast:

> Interestingly, immature hepatocytes (9–25 weeks' gestation) were also positive for all three enzymes . . . This finding suggests that the three enzymes transiently appear in immature hepatocytes during the fetal period and that they are secreted from immature hepatocytes into the blood stream via the sinusoids and/or into bile ducts via bile canaliculi. Therefore, it seems likely that fetal primitive hilar bile ducts and hepatocytes are among the cellular sources of these enzymes during the fetal period.[81]

One must suspect, as did Beard, that these enzymes evident so early in development, long before any digestive requirement, must fulfill some need essential to the well-being, even the survival, of the developing embryo. Why else would there be two sources and not just one?

Beard 100 years ago knew nothing of such hepatic synthesis of embryonic "pancreatic" enzymes, but the evidence does confirm what he long ago proposed, that these "ferments" including trypsin do appear at least by week 8–9.

Carlson sums up the more recent evidence suggesting the early production of enzymes, some time before week 8.[4(pp338-340)] He reports that the pancreas begins forming during the fifth week after conception as two distinct and separate buds, the larger dorsal and the smaller ventral pancreas, each arising from the foregut, the forerunner of the intestinal tract. Even at this stage, some quantity of the enzymes appears in the primitive pancreatic acinar cells, though admittedly in very small amounts. By the seventh week, when the two segments have migrated into their final position in the retroperitoneal space and at the same time, fused together, enzyme levels increase, just as Beard reported. After 8 weeks, their synthesis stabilizes for a time, before skyrocketing at 6–7 months.[4(p338-339)]

It is also important to consider that during fetal life, pancreatic enzymes such as trypsin and its precursor trypsinogen percolate into the trophoblastic tissues not only from the embryo, but also from the mother via the uterine circulation. Physiologists have known for decades that in adult humans our blood contains all the major pancreatic enzymes, and laboratories have long provided normal ranges for each.[82] During pancreatitis, blood levels of the enzymes increase dramatically, followed by a drop back to normal with improvement.

Colombo makes reference to the routine appearance of pancreatic enzymes in the blood of adults:

> Pancreatic enzymes are normally present in the blood in very low concentrations as a probable result of a direct passage from the pancreas through the ductal and acinovenous system. With the availability of sensitive and specific analytic techniques, determination of serum immunoreactive trypsin(ogen) (IRT) has proven useful in the assessment of pancreatic dysfunction that may occur in a variety of clinical conditions, and IRT assay on dried blood spot is the most reliable test of screening for cystic fibrosis.[80]

Conventional physiologists have never proposed any purpose for these pancreatic secretions circulating in all of us. But, with nature being conservative and biologically thrifty, one would logically expect that if molecules such as trypsin routinely appear in our blood, they must be there for a reason. Perhaps they fill the role proposed by Beard, serving as our main protection against cancer—and in the pregnant woman, as regulators of trophoblast growth.

In an earlier chapter, when we reviewed the physiology and molecular biology of the trophoblast, we reported that during the initial weeks after conception, before any of the differentiated tissues appear, the outer layer of the trophoblast furthest away from the inner cell mass, the syncytiotrophoblast, transforms first into a collection of noninvasive giant cells.[8] Only later does the trophoblast tissue nearest the developing embryo, at a time its pancreas would be forming, follow suit, morphing itself into a highly differentiated and non-aggressive tissue.

If Beard's hypothesis holds true, that proteolytic pancreatic enzymes regulate trophoblast destiny, then at first glance this chronology might make little sense. However, the syncytiotrophoblast tissues furthest from the inner cell mass, hence most distant from the embryo body, would be in closest contact with the maternal blood and its complement of enzymes, as they travel through the placental tissues. Perhaps the mother's contribution sets off the process of trophoblast maturation, before the synthetic apparatus in the embryonic pancreas turns on sufficiently. When fetal production of enzymes subsequently begins, we would expect the trophoblast nearest the embryo then to transform into a more differentiated tissue, just as is observed.

We have now shown that contemporary investigators confirmed the presence of enzymes within the embryonic pancreas at about the time Beard claimed, 7–8 weeks. But, we need to address the second pertinent point: Does the change of the invasive trophoblast into the mature placenta truly coincide with their initial synthesis?

As we now know, the metamorphosis of the trophoblastic tissues, their evolution into the complex placenta, occurs gradually, beginning shortly after the trophoblast and inner cell mass proceed along their separate developmental pathways. For the first 8 weeks after conception, before the placenta takes final form, the fledgling embryo must obtain the nutrients and oxygen it needs for survival by diffusion through the decidua of the uterus. By week 8 the placenta assumes its basic shape and structure, and between week 8 and week 12, the organ reaches full maturity, with its complex blood circulation firmly established and functional.[14;83(p946)] So the transition from the undifferentiated, invasive trophoblast of early pregnancy into the highly differentiated non-invasive placenta occurs about the time Beard predicted, commencing about seven to eight weeks after conception, just as embryonic production of trypsin and other proteolytic enzymes, within both the pancreas and hepato-biliary system, turns on in earnest.

# CHAPTER 9

# The Evolution of Enzyme Treatment

During his lifetime, Dr. Beard recommended only injectable preparations of pancreatic enzymes as a cancer treatment. For his specific purposes, he assumed orally ingested preparations would be of little value. The active components such as trypsin are proteins, and like any other protein ingested by mouth would face a series of formidable barriers, beginning with the hydrochloric acid present in the stomach. Any active enzymes that might survive this initial assault would then be subjected to auto-digestion within the alkaline duodenum. Should any trypsin remain, it could do little systemically; scientists at the time already knew the protease to be a fairly large molecule that, they believed, could not possibly pass through the intestinal mucosa.

In Beard's day, a number of pharmaceutical firms in Europe and in the US manufactured powdered enzyme products, designed as a treatment for diphtheria, a world-wide scourge until the advent of vaccines for the disease. The diphtheria bacillus killed its host by elaborating a tough fibrous membrane in the throat that could, if unchecked, lead to suffocation. In an animal model of the disease, a preparation of trypsin locally applied in the larynx appeared to dissolve this deadly tissue and when tested in humans, the enzyme worked quite well. An early reference to the successful treatment in humans dates from the October 23, 1886 issue of the *Journal of the American Medical Association*.[84]

By 1900, two companies, Merck and the New York based Fairchild, affiliated with Burroughs Wellcome, marketed trypsin preparations derived from animal sources for treatment of the disease. An old catalogue of Fairchild we have uncovered from 1898 lists, as one of its products: "TRYPSIN. (FAIRCHILD.) ESPECIALLY PREPARED AS A SOLVENT FOR DIPHTHERITIC MEMBRANE."[85(p57)] It seems around that time, companies such as Fairchild began marketing injectable preparations in addition to those intended for direct application.

By 1907, the initial successes reported in the literature generated considerable interest in Beard's enzyme treatment of cancer. In response to this enthusiasm, a growing number of firms began selling their own "trypsin" specifically as a cancer treatment in addition to those available from Merck and Fairchild. With trypsin formulations widely available, physicians both in the US and in Europe began applying the therapy, usually without consulting Beard, and with variable results. As both positive and negative reports began to filter into the literature, Beard began to suspect that many of the available preparations had little potency and hence, little efficacy. He himself, after testing various products, recommended only the enzymes available from Fairchild, which he thought most effective clinically.[86]

Manufacturers of pancreatic enzymes in those days faced numerous difficulties bringing a potent formulation to market. Then, as now, all commercial enzymes were extracted from the glands of animals, such as cattle and pigs, slaughtered for their meat. In the animal pancreas, the acinar cells synthesize and store the proteolytic components as inactive precursors such as trypsinogen and chymotrypsinogen, to protect the gland itself. During meals, in response to both hormonal and neural stimulus, the exocrine cells release their supply of inactive proteases directly into the pancreatic ducts. The ductal cells themselves secrete a bicarbonate-rich fluid, which along with the enzymes ultimately empties into the duodenum (small intestine). Since the proteolytic component works best in a slightly alkaline pH, the accompanying bicarbonate neutralizes any acid arriving from the stomach during digestion, and in so doing creates the ideal environment for the enzymes to begin their work.

In the duodenum the intestinal enzyme enterokinase secreted by the mucosal cells cleaves off a small six amino acid terminal from trypsinogen, converting the precursor into the active enzyme.[11(p227)] Trypsin can then rapidly begin activating other trypsinogen and chymotrypsinogen molecules in a cascade effect.

At room temperature in the presence of even small amounts of moisture, the precursors can begin spontaneously converting into active enzymes, even in the absence of enterokinase. After only a few trypsin molecules so transform, these can then rapidly set off the activation process. Consequently, in an animal pancreas sitting in a slaughterhouse waiting to be collected for drug company use, all the enzymes can convert into the active configuration unless cooled on ice and processed very quickly. Since trypsin and chymotrypsin are themselves proteins, the potent enzymes can begin attacking one another, rendering the mixture into a collection of inert peptide fragments and amino acids.

From our readings in the literature, it seems that in Beard's era, the manufacturers used a very simple process to extract the enzymes, first mincing the glands in cold water, pressing the mixture, then removing the active component with alcohol. The alcohol would then be allowed to evaporate off, leaving the desired enzyme fraction.[87]

We suspect the procedure was neither exacting nor refined, the final preparation most likely containing little in the way of potential enzyme activity. To make matters worse, those products intended for injectable use were provided in an aqueous solution in vial form, an ideal environment for the auto-digestion process to begin. Fairchild did market a dry powdered "trypsin" meant to be mixed with water immediately before injection, but even this proved so unstable that by 1907, as Beard reports, the company discontinued its sale.[3]

In the November 16, 1907 issue of *Lancet,* P. Tetens Hald, M.D., "Formerly Assistant in the Pharmacological Institute of the University of Copenhagen" and a Beard proponent, published the results of his evaluation of six popular enzyme products available at the time, including those marketed by Merck and Fairchild.[88] In his research, he employed the same method used today to assess proteolytic activity, the casein digestion test. This simple assay measures the amount of the milk protein casein curdled over time by a known quantity of pancreas product. Today, laboratories measure enzymatic potency much the same way, rating activity with a 1-10X USP system, in which each unit signifies the product has digested 25 times its weight of casein. So, a gram of a "1X" product can digest 25 grams of casein, a gram of a "4X" product, 100 grams, and so on.

Dr. Hald contacted the manufacturers of the various products he analyzed in his laboratory, none of whom provided him with any information about the stability of the formulations they sold commercially. To his surprise, his assays revealed the potencies varied enormously, up to a factor of 400, and that the activity levels rarely correlated with the company's claims, as stated on the bottle or in its literature.

Dr. Hald writes:

> The results are interesting in several respects. First, they show that preparations obtained from different makers vary exceedingly in strength. Thus the strongest of the preparations examined was 400 times more active than the weakest one. The feeble action of the preparations obtained from Zanoni and from Freund and Redlich was very striking. . .
>
> Secondly, Table III shows that even the preparations of the same class may present considerable differences in strength. In one brand one of the supplies was even between 30 and 40 times stronger than the other one . . .[88]

In his 1911 book *The Enzyme Treatment of Cancer*, Dr. Beard himself bemoaned the dearth of standardized and potent enzyme preparations, a situation that led to inevitable treatment failures when physicians utilized products of poor quality. He actually quotes a Merck publication from the time, in which the writer discusses the confusion in the field:

> The actual position of affairs in the past few years can best be described by quoting the impartial opinion of a competent author. On p. 340 of *E. Merck's Annual Report of Recent Advances in Pharmaceutical Chemistry and Therapeutics* (Darmstadt, vol. xxii., August, 1909) one may read regarding trypsin: "The mode of action and the value of pancreas preparations

in cancer has not yet received a wholly reliable explanation. Great difficulties are encountered because the preparations used by the various investigators differ greatly in respect to their chemical properties, their purity, and in the amount of active substances they contain, and often these factors are not fully known to the student of the literature, or to the physician who has used them and describes their action. Further difficulties arise when pancreatin [whole pancreas product] and trypsin are described as substances of equal value, and how shall we gauge the action of pancreatin and trypsin ampullae whose mode of preparation and whose composition is not mentioned in the original paper, neither is there any mention made of their sterility or the method by which they have been sterilized? . . . So long as the solutions of pancreatin and trypsin are treated as secret remedies no one will be able to form a clear picture of the value of trypsin treatment from the many publications which have appeared."[3(p198)]

In reference to the above, as an aside we find it interesting that by 1909 Beard's hypothesis had generated interest sufficient enough to warrant thoughtful discussion in the annual report of a major international pharmaceutical company. The above exposition also adds support to Beard's contention that the mixed results for enzyme treatment being reported in the literature most likely reflected no flaw in the theory, only variations in the quality of product.

A number of factors contributed to the decline of interest after 1911 in Dr. Beard's trophoblastic hypothesis and his enzyme approach to cancer. Certainly, the enthusiasm for the X-ray, discovered in 1895 by Röntgen, helped push Beard's treatment into the background.[89;90] After all, two-time Nobel Laureate Madame Curie, widely admired and respected at all levels of society, had vigorously championed the mysterious invisible rays as a non-toxic cure for all cancer, a breakthrough the press promoted with great enthusiasm. Beard had no such media savvy science star to praise his esoteric ideas about the fish blastoderm, the trophoblast, the germ cell spore, and the use of enzymes against malignant disease. And it would not be until after Beard's death in 1924 that researchers began to appreciate the severe limitations of radiation treatment, which in reality worked well against only a few cancers. Even for those tumors that did respond initially, usually the disease recurred with a vengeance and the therapy once thought to be harmless actually could be quite toxic. An entire generation of radiation researchers died as a result of cavalier exposure to the rays, including Madame Curie herself who eventually succumbed to radiation-induced aplastic anemia.[91] By then, Beard was long forgotten.

Above and beyond the influence of personality, the vagaries of the media, and the realities of scientific politics, we suspect that poor quality enzyme products did much to undermine Beard's treatment. In a sense, Beard was a victim of his own fame. The initial successes reported in the literature prompted many doctors to begin using any number of enzyme formulations without first consulting Beard about dosing and quality, with inevitable poor or mixed results. The disappointments fueled the backlash in the journals, to the point that after 1911, few doctors of Beard's generation even considered the treatment for their patients.[74]

Subsequently, F.L. Morse, M.D. in St. Louis during the late 1920s and early 1930s,[92] and Frank Shively, M.D., a Dayton, Ohio surgeon active during the 1960s,[93] rediscovered Beard's earlier papers and used injectable formulations of the pancreatic enzymes in their treatment protocols with reported success. Then in the 1960s, William Kelley, D.D.S. first appeared on the scene, with his complex cancer treatment involving a whole foods diet, large amounts of various nutritional supplements, detoxification routines, and prodigious doses of pancreatic enzymes ingested orally—but never injected.

Kelley claimed he discovered the anti-cancer properties of oral pancreatic enzymes serendipitously, without any apparent previous knowledge of Dr. Beard. Kelley had been a successful orthodontist with a serious interest in nutrition, practicing in Grapevine, Texas, when in the early 1960s while he was only in his mid-30s, he became devastatingly ill. His doctors eventually diagnosed advanced pancreatic cancer, though he never underwent tissue sampling—not uncommon in the days before CT scans and needle biopsies. In desperation, with four children dependent on him, Kelley devised his own nutritional program to slow the disease, including a largely organic, vegetarian raw foods type diet, a variety of supplements, and detoxification routines such as coffee enemas. He also added high doses of oral pancreatic enzymes to his regimen, not because of any familiarity with Beard's trophoblastic hypothesis of which he was at the time ignorant, but to help relieve his severe digestive distress—as occurs commonly in patients with pancreatic malignancy.

Kelley's digestion was so poor, he began ingesting huge amounts of pancreatin around the clock hoping to keep his worsening symptoms—including excruciating pain whenever he ate—at bay. He discovered that with large doses, his tolerance for food improved and—to his surprise—his large tumors, palpable through the abdominal wall, seemed to regress. Perplexed, and ever the serious student, he scoured the medical literature looking for evidence that someone else might have observed an anti-cancer effect for the pancreatic enzymes. His search eventually led him to Dr. Beard's book and papers from 50 years earlier, but by that point, Kelley claimed, he had already worked out the rudiments of his treatment.

From that very personal experience began Kelley's foray out of conventional orthodontics into the controversial world of nutritional cancer therapeutics. By the late 1960s, having long abandoned dentistry, he refocused his attention on treating, with his nutritional regimen, the very ill drawn from all over the country, most diagnosed with advanced malignancy. With the publication of his 1969 book *One Answer to Cancer*,[94] Kelley for better or worse secured his position as a preeminent alternative cancer therapist, and inevitably as a target for the mainstream medical world which then, as now, had little use for proposed nutritional approaches to the disease.

Kelley intently studied the writings of Beard, who strongly insisted the treatment needed to be applied via injection. Nonetheless, for the duration of his career, Kelley only recommended oral formulations. Injectable preparations were still available in the US until 1966, when the FDA in its wisdom enacted a regulation removing them from the marketplace, perhaps in response to Dr. Shively's practice. In any event, as a dentist, Kelley lacked the legal right to prescribe injectable enzymes, so the question was moot. Most importantly, even if such products remained available and even if he had the authority to use them, his own experience treating himself, and his subsequent experience with hundreds of patients taught him that oral preparations worked very well despite Beard's claims to the contrary.

From the early 1900s, oral formulations of pancreatic enzymes were available with and without prescription in the US and Europe for a variety of uses, including treatment for diphtheria as well as digestive problems. Dr. Rice, who published the first report we have been able to identify of a patient successfully treated with enzymes, recommended the Fairchild injectable preparation along with an oral supplement known as "Holadin."[69] In the decades that followed, physicians prescribed these oral products for their patients diagnosed with pancreatic insufficiency such as occurs with pancreatitis or cystic fibrosis, though no one until Kelley used them as a primary cancer treatment.

By 1950, the commercial demand for pancreatic enzymes such as trypsin had expanded greatly beyond their limited pharmaceutical application. For example, leather tanners used proteolytic enzymes to speed up curing, and candy manufacturers learned that trypsin, when added during the processing of chocolate, helped create a smoother product.

But the commercial suppliers still relied on the old mincing and alcohol method of extracting proteolytic enzymes from the animal gland, a very inefficient technique that gave a 10–15% yield.[87] A potential bonanza awaited anyone who might develop a more efficient enzyme purification process.

The biochemist Ezra Levin of Champaign, Illinois, active during the 1940s and 1950s and at the time one of the leading experts in the manufacture of pancreatic enzymes, believed he had done just that. His lengthy 1950 US patent entitled *Production of Dried, Defatted Enzymatic Material* detailed his crowning achievement, an elaborate multi-step process for extracting active enzymes from the gland that he insisted was more efficient and more cost effective than the previous methodology.[87] Instead of removing a portion of the enzymes from the pancreas tissue, leaving most behind in the discarded residue, Levin's new method involved first extracting the fat with appropriate solvents.

Then any remaining water would be evaporated off via vacuum distillation, leaving all the enzymes in the remaining powder that yielded, at least theoretically, a very potent product.[87] In a sense, Levin had reversed the traditional procedure in which the enzymes were extracted from the pancreatic tissue, with the water, fat, and most of the enzymes remaining behind as waste.

Levin saw as an added benefit that during the process, most if not all the precursors such as trypsinogen would also simultaneously activate, to yield a product of high potency with purported minimal processing losses—a product which Levin and his customers thought most ideal for pharmaceutical as well as industrial use.

Levin had made two assumptions, as he perfected his method. First, he believed that the fat in the gland—and the pancreas is a fatty gland—had no useful purpose beyond its role as a storage depot for excess calories, and needed to be removed. To him, fat seemed little more than inert filler. Second, he always assumed the more activated the product, the better.

On the first page of his patent, an introductory summary of his method reflects his two basic assumptions:

> By the present invention, trypsinogen is converted to trypsin and chymotrypsinogen to chymotrypsin by pre-activation to a maximum and is then dried and defatted simultaneously as hereinafter described, while this high enzymatic activity is held substantially without change, to produce highly active raw powders equal in activity to the fresh gland.[87]

Levin actually created a company, Viobin, for years a subsidiary of A.H. Robbins, to manufacture and market his enzyme products. The Levin method proved so successful that by the 1960s, Viobin provided most of the enzymes used in the US, both for pharmaceutical and other industrial purposes. Even other manufacturers that ventured into the enzyme business themselves relied on variations of the Levin patent.

Throughout the 1970s, Kelley designed his own extensive line of supplements, produced by a number of different companies. At one point, he told me he had gone through 14 such firms in 20 years, changing when he felt quality control failed to meet his standards, which in the supplement industry in those days tended to be lax. However, whatever company name might appear on the label, Kelley insisted the pancreatic raw material be purchased from Viobin, which he always claimed to be the best available enzyme. The various distributors he used would purchase the pancreatin in bulk powdered form and encapsulate the material, with the final product bottled and distributed under Kelley's personal label. Even though other suppliers approached him, for all of Dr. Kelley's 20 years in practice as a nutritional therapist, he stuck by Viobin through the years of his great success and his growing reputation.

The Levin method could be adjusted, by shortening or lengthening the processing time, to provide pancreatin of various potencies as measured on the 1-10X scale, with 1X representing the least, and 10X, the maximum possible activity. During the 1970s, Viobin actually sold pancreatin of various activity levels, a number of which Kelley tried out over the years. Eventually, after vacillating back and forth from weaker to stronger then back to weaker formulations, he settled for a time on the 4X which provided more than half of the total potential enzyme content as inactive precursors.

By the time I (Dr. Gonzalez) met Kelley during the summer of 1981, he had become convinced that the more active the oral product, the better the effect against cancer. He wanted 8-10X, nothing less, for all his patients. He seemed at times almost fanatical about the issue of enzyme strength, insisting he wanted no precursors in his formulation. I even travelled with Kelley to Wisconsin to meet with the manufacturer he used at the time, to discuss with them his new plans for the strongest supplement possible, containing only 10X pancreatin. I also met several times with representatives of Viobin, to discuss their enzymes and the feasibility of providing large amounts of the 10X material.

As I pursued my investigation of Dr. Kelley's therapy and practice over the next five years under my mentor, the late Robert A. Good, M.D., Ph.D., I concentrated my efforts primarily on Kelley's results with advanced cancer. As a side project, I also tried to evaluate the relative efficacy of the different pancreatic formulations he had recommended during his time in practice. From Kelley's records and our conversations about the issue, I had a fairly good idea of which strength of enzyme he used during which period.

From my review of Kelley's patient records on a year by year basis, it seemed to me that his greatest success as a practitioner occurred during the decade 1970–1980, when he relied primarily on the 4X pancreatin, containing a high percentage of inactive precursors. After 1981, he opted for increasingly more activated product, eventually settling on the 10X potency. However, it appeared that his success declined markedly as he prescribed a "stronger" preparation. Admittedly, other factors might have come into play: beginning in 1981, Kelley himself withdrew from direct patient care, turning his therapy over to a constellation of "Kelley Counselors" whom he had trained via a series of weekend seminars. Though he had over the years certified over 1000 such practitioners, only several dozen were active at the time I met Kelley, and these consisted of a very mixed group of people, in both educational background and ability. Some were practicing physicians, dentists, and chiropractors, others had no professional education in health care whatsoever. While a number I found to be very competent and dedicated, including several who lacked formal medical training, many were far less so. It would be hard to sort out the influence of this dramatic shift in the administration of his program on its successful application.

Regardless of the cause, I could track a significant fall off in responders beginning about 1982—in fact, during the years 1984–1985, as I actively brought my research to a close, I knew of only one impressive result, a patient with stage IV Hodgkin's disease whose cancer regressed completely on the enzyme therapy. This single success during that time represented a far different situation than Kelley's glory days of the 1970s when, by my investigation of his charts, many hundreds of patients with properly diagnosed cancer had done well. But this patient was to my knowledge the last great success, and by 1986, Kelley in great frustration had closed his organization, essentially cutting off his treatment after 20 years. He believed that "disloyal" counselors and greedy supplement manufacturers had effectively sabotaged his life's work.

I finished my project under Dr. Good in 1986, but sadly Kelley turned increasingly paranoid, at one point thinking I had been sent by the CIA to steal his therapy for the government. After 1987, I had no further direct contact with Kelley, who for a long time essentially disappeared from view.

When Dr. Isaacs and I subsequently arrived in New York in the fall of 1987 determined to salvage Kelley's treatment, we knew if we were to succeed in practice, we needed a reliable source of enzymes. As I thought about the situation, I realized we must determine the optimal composition for the enzyme product in terms of relative fat and protein content, as well as the ideal level of proteolytic activity—and hopefully find a source that met our specifications.

I had already begun to move away from the Levin methodology as the best for manufacturing pancreatic enzymes. In terms of composition, I knew that he had designed his extraction method to remove as much fat as possible, which he perceived as useless filler. I thought in this regard Levin, as well as Kelley, who accepted without question Levin's dictates, had been wrong, that fat might allow for a more stable product and provide physiological benefit. By 1987, researchers had already begun to suspect that fat was not just a simple warehouse for storing excess energy, but a metabolically active tissue secreting a variety of enzymes and hormones that regulate the processing of sugars and fatty acids. Perhaps, I thought, the lipid component of the pancreas might itself provide some additional effect, a complement to the proteolytic activity. So as a first order of business, I decided to search for an enzyme preparation containing significant fat.

Ezra Levin also assumed that the more active the product the better, the mantra Kelley again professed to me with total conviction. But I knew from my exhaustive evaluation of Kelley's files that as he opted for a more potent enzyme formulation, his response rate fell significantly. In frustration, he assumed he only needed to prescribe an even stronger enzyme, or change encapsulators, etc., instead of retracing his steps and going backward to the less active 4X enzymes he had earlier used with great success.

I became convinced that as brilliant as Kelley had been in his prime, he had erred in his later years by assuming that "purer and stronger" is always unquestionably better. I suspected that the fat depleted, highly activated supplements may have been prone to deteriorate once encapsulated, susceptible to rapid auto-digestion on the shelf. That may have been part of Kelley's problem during the mid-1980s. I also became convinced that the fat in the gland might not only help stabilize the mix, but provide synergistic factors to assist the proteolytic enzymes in their fight against malignant cells. Finally, I came to believe that an enzyme with less activity, with more of the total potential as precursor, might not only be more stable in the bottle, but more effective against cancer.

As a first order of business, I obtained samples of pancreatin from a number of suppliers who manufactured their own products. I also visited several health food stores and nutritional pharmacies in Manhattan, such as Willner's, purchasing a variety of pancreatic enzyme supplements. In the kitchen of my mother's home in Queens where we were staying at the time, I set up my own enzyme assay, using Knox gelatin as my protein substrate instead of casein, and the Viobin preparation Viokase as my standard by which to measure the activity of other products. I dissolved each capsule or tablet in a slightly alkaline solution to help promote the enzymatic reactions, and then observed the amount of gelatin digested over time. The assay, which I repeated many times over a number of weeks, worked quite well. Unfortunately, nearly all of the enzymes I tested seemed highly activated and highly processed, with all the fat removed.

Finally, I learned of the pancreas enzyme product derived from New Zealand pigs available from Allergy Research Group, a nutritional supplement company of some renown based in Northern California. As a start, I was happy about the source, since I had learned that New Zealand had perhaps the cleanest environment of any country on earth, as well as the strictest laws for raising animals for commercial use. Diseases such as hoof and mouth disease and trichinosis, I was told, had never been reported there.

I also wanted enzymes derived from the pig pancreas, thought to be most similar to the human organ. For decades, before the advent of genetically engineered preparations, physicians treated their diabetic patients with pig insulin, which proved to be quite similar in terms of amino acid structure to the human variety. In a similar manner, pig enzymes, I had learned from my conversations with Viobin scientists, most closely resembled ours, of all commercially available sources.

Most importantly, the Allergy Research Group (ARG) specifications described their pancreas supplement as a freeze dried product, minimally processed, *with the fat intact*, yet it still tested active at moderate levels by my own assay—exactly what we wanted. Though the material had not been intentionally activated as per Levin, I suspected during the handling of the glands, some of the precursors spontaneously converted, fortuitously to the precise level we thought ideal. Then, with freeze drying complete, all activation would come to a halt, leaving a stable product with most of the proteolytic enzymes in the precursor form.

I contacted the founder of ARG, Dr. Stephen Levine, and introduced myself, explaining my plan to open up a practice and my need for good quality enzymes. Though I was virtually unknown at the time, he agreed to provide me with as much of the product as we required. With a supply of enzymes guaranteed, in late 1987 we opened our practice with great optimism in an office in Manhattan. To our relief, this enzyme worked quite well, confirming my belief that a minimally processed lightly activated preparation, with the fat intact, was ideal for our purposes. One of my first successes dated from December 1987, a woman diagnosed with inflammatory breast cancer who had developed metastases into the bone while receiving chemotherapy. Told she had terminal disease, she somehow learned about us and began our program. She is alive today, over 21 years later, in excellent health with all scans long ago showing complete regression of her disease.

We treated all our early successes, right up until 1995, with pancreatic enzymes available from ARG. Between 1995 and 1998, we entered into a research and development arrangement with Procter & Gamble, who generously provided extensive financial support as well as a team of scientists to help us determine definitively the best enzyme formulation for our purposes. The company spent considerable time, effort, and money evaluating our enzymes, even sending researchers to New Zealand to observe first hand the entire processing of the pancreas glands from slaughterhouse to finished material. With such assistance, we eventually refined the methodology still further, to help guarantee consistent manufacture of a stable, modestly active, minimally processed product with most of the enzymes—but not all—in the precursor form, and with a certain percentage of fat remaining. Working with our New Zealand supplier, we developed a method to help assure the desired potency with each batch, without the need for Levin's complicated system of fat extraction and vacuum distillation. Today, we still rely on that same enzyme preparation, which we find works even more effectively than our earlier supplement.

# CHAPTER 10

# Oral Versus Injectable Preparations

I n his classic 1897 text *Collected Contributions on Digestion and Diet*, the English physiologist Sir William Roberts reported his experiments "proving" that hydrochloric acid permanently inactivated pancreatic "ferments," as he called the enzymes.[65(p47)] As a result of his laboratory work, Roberts concluded orally ingested preparations of enzymes would be of little benefit as digestive aids, or for any other purpose. Beard knew of Roberts' writings which he held in some esteem, even referencing him by name in his own book *The Enzyme Treatment of Cancer*.[3(p201)] Fully accepting Roberts' conclusions, Beard insisted that for any effect against cancer, the practitioner must administer the pancreas enzymes in an injectable form. Though Beard's proponents such as Dr. Rice did prescribe oral preparations along with the injectable, these were intended strictly as supplemental, not as primary therapy.[69]

Today, 100 years later, most physiologists still cite the same mantra proposed by Roberts, claiming that pancreatic enzymes ingested orally cannot survive contact with hydrochloric acid in the stomach. Even if they did somehow escape acid destruction, the teaching goes that in the alkaline small intestine they would be subject to auto-digestion, rendering the enzymes into inert protein fragments. Supposing, hypothetically of course, some enzymes might endure this second attack unscathed, in no way could these large complex molecules then be absorbed through the intestinal wall into the circulation for systemic effect against cancer or any other disease. Critics of our work proclaim that even if pancreatic enzymes do have an anti-cancer potential, our therapy as administered today can't possibly succeed because we prescribe oral formulations exclusively. When I lecture, usually at the end someone will question the feasibility of systemic benefit with the oral supplements we recommend.

With all due respect to Dr. Beard, physiologists, and critics, orally ingested pancreatic enzymes must survive digestive assault and be absorbed because in practice they work, as Kelley's successes and our own would attest. But such a response does not answer the legitimate scientific questions asked regarding the efficacy of oral preparations. If we put aside Kelley's experience or ours for a moment, a review of the scientific literature does not support the current dogma, but long ago confirmed that pancreatic enzymes taken by mouth survive the gauntlet of the digestive tract and can be absorbed into the systemic circulation to a substantial degree.

The late physician Dr. Edward Howell first investigated in some depth the absorption of orally ingested enzymes for possible therapeutic action during the first half of the 20th century. Howell was not an academic scientist, but a practicing physician and independent researcher, best known as the grandfather of the current raw foods movement. Howell proposed decades ago that raw foodstuffs provide all the vitamins, minerals, trace elements, fibers, proteins, fats, and carbohydrates in an undamaged, optimal form allowing for greatest physiological benefit. Among these essentials he also included enzymes present in our food, which he believed could be absorbed intact and active like a vitamin or mineral, to aid in normal metabolism and in repair of tissue damage.

Raw food contains multiple classes of enzymes in its constituent cells, as part of their normal biochemical and metabolic machinery. However, with temperatures above 117°F, these "food enzymes," as Howell called them, generally denature. Cooking therefore not only destroys certain vitamins such as folate and renders certain minerals such as calcium less available for use, but categorically, Howell believed, inactivates all food enzymes. Much disease, Howell in turn proposed, results from our dependence on a largely cooked, nutrient and enzyme depleted diet.

In his clinical practice, Howell applied a variety of raw foods diets and enzyme supplements, claiming great success. Judging by his writings, he became rather expert not only in dietetics, but in the field of enzymes, their therapeutic use, and particularly, their absorption when taken by mouth. In his 1946 book, *The Status of Food Enzymes in Digestion and Metabolism*, later reprinted as *Food Enzymes for Health & Longevity*,[95] he reviewed the literature on enzyme therapeutics to that time. Surprisingly enough he seems to have been totally ignorant of Dr. Beard's thesis from 40 years earlier.

Despite that oversight, in a chapter entitled "Intestinal Absorbability of Enzymes," Dr. Howell argues the case from the scientific literature that pancreatic enzymes specifically ingested as supplements survive digestion to be absorbed from the intestinal tract into both the bloodstream as well as the lymphatic system.[95(pp12-23)]

His well-referenced document, though old, makes interesting reading from a historical perspective. When I (Dr. Gonzalez) first studied the book, I was surprised to learn that even by 1946, a considerable body of evidence indicated large proteins in general, and pancreatic enzymes in particular, taken by mouth did end up in the general circulation. In the following, Howell discusses the findings from a group of Japanese researchers who evaluated the levels of enzymes in urine over a 24 hour period after an oral challenge:

> What I believe is one of the most outstanding researches so far recorded on the fate of enzymes when taken orally was undertaken by Masumizu, Medical Clinic, Tohoku Imperial University, Japan. Masumizu's work is remarkable in several ways. The experiments were conducted, not upon isolated specimens of urine, but upon the complete 24 hour excretion, thereby insuring the presence of all enzymes excreted, instead of only a portion. The experimental animals, 10 rabbits, were given by os [mouth], 5 grams of pancreatin or 5 grams of fungus amylase for each rabbit per day. Since this dosage is comparatively enormous for small animals, the experiments prove beyond doubt that even large quantities of enzymes can be absorbed and find their way into the urine.

> Although Masumizu proved that the urinary excretion of amylase was approximately doubled when the enzymes were given, he was unable to secure any increase in the serum amylase concentration at all. He remarks that in all his experiments the level of amylase in the serum always remained constant and his figures bear out this contention. This confirms the observation of Oelgoetz who likewise found the serum amylase level uninfluenced by ingested enzymes . . . [95(pp12-13)]

As an aside to the above, in his book Howell argues that the stable serum levels of amylase observed say nothing about its absorption. He believed most animals have intricate mechanisms to keep blood levels of such enzymes within a fairly narrow range, quickly sending excess into tissues for storage.

In more recent times, the published literature again confirms that orally ingested enzymes can survive exposure to hydrochloric acid in the stomach, the alkaline environment of the duodenum, and be absorbed efficiently through the small intestinal mucosa.

Using more contemporary documentation, we will address these issues beginning with the alleged inactivation of pancreatic enzymes by hydrochloric acid in the gut, a chronic refrain over the years. Many of the reports making this claim date to the 1970s and 1980s: for example, in a *New England Journal of Medicine* article published in 1977, Regan et al discuss the clinical efficacy of pancreatic enzyme preparations, administered along with acid neutralizing medications. They write, in their introduction:

> Oral pancreatic extracts are employed routinely in treatment for the malabsorption that occurs in pancreatic insufficiency . . . Some patients remain symptomatic, with diarrhea, and fail to gain weight. In vitro and in vivo observations suggest that this therapeutic failure is due to inactivation of lipase and trypsin by gastric acid and pepsin. Therefore, we investigated the efficacy of various adjunctive measures in protecting the activity of orally ingested enzymes.[96]

In a later article published in 1979 entitled "An Enteric-Coated Pancreatic Enzyme Preparation that Works," the authors discuss their experiences with a new oral enzyme product specifically designed to survive the alleged insurmountable obstacle of stomach acid. They write:

> The hostile acid environment of the stomach acts as a formidable barrier though which pH-sensitive enzymes must proceed. A variety of methods have been utilized in attempts to overcome this barrier, including neutralization and/or inhibition of gastric acid secretion and the use of enteric-coated preparations.[97]

In a 1982 report appearing in *Gastroenterology*, Dutta and colleagues detail their evaluation of enteric-coated enzyme preparations. In their introduction, they write:

> Medical treatment of patients with pancreatic insufficiency is generally less than satisfactory because of persistent steatorrhea on treatment with large doses of pancreatic enzyme supplements. Inactivation of orally ingested pancreatic enzyme by gastric acid is considered to be a major factor responsible for inadequate response to enzyme therapy in this group of patients.[98]

In a more recent 1989 article entitled "Theory and Practice in the Individualization of Oral Pancreatic Enzyme Administration for Chronic Pancreatitis," the authors repeat the same refrain:

> Gastric acid plays a role in malabsorption, since administered enzymes may be destroyed by gastric acid.[99]

Despite the above claims, even a cursory review of the actual scientific literature shows pancreatic proteolytic enzymes, particularly trypsin, very nicely survive the supposed ravages of stomach acid. An article by Moskvichyov et al of the All-Union Scientific Research Technological Institute of Antibiotics and Enzymes for Medical Applications published in *Enzyme Microbiology and Technology* in 1988 discusses this very issue in some detail.[100]

In their article, the authors begin by reviewing the previously published data, which rather conclusively demonstrated the stability of trypsin exposed to high temperatures even in the presence of acid:

> In the first reports by J.H. Northrop, J. Mellanby and V.J. Woolley on heating trypsin in dilute acid solutions up to boiling point it was demonstrated that activity loss was minimal. The unusual property of trypsin, i.e. its high thermostability, was not clearly understood then. The most interesting and promising reports did not appear until the late 1960s, when the kinetics of the reverse denaturation of trypsin and chymotrypsin were described. It was then established that the unusual properties of these proteinases are due to the conformational transitions between different states of the protein molecule while the equilibrium between them may shift, depending upon external conditions.[100]

In terms of its documented heat stability, trypsin does seem unique among enzymes, certainly far different in character than the thermolabile "food enzymes" described by Howell.

Moskvichyov and colleagues describe their own elaborate experiments proving stability of trypsin even when exposed to acid at high temperatures. The authors demonstrated that in a solution of heated acid, active trypsin exists in a dynamic equilibrium with its denatured configuration. With higher heat and greater acid concentration, the reaction favors the denatured form; with cooling and a more alkaline pH, the process yields more of the active trypsin. In this system, the inactive conformation, apparently protected from damage, can convert, as pH goes up and temperature drops, back into the functional enzyme. This work proves that trypsin denaturation by heat or acid is *not permanent, but a reversible process*—thus contradicting the basic assumptions of many.

Therefore, orally ingested pancreatic enzyme preparations should easily survive the hydrochloric acid present in the stomach. In the next assumed obstacle, the alkaline liquid environment of the duodenum, the enzymes become most active—and most susceptible, the experts teach, to auto-digestion. Few of these molecules, they claim, could possibly survive this drive to mass molecular suicide.

Once again, contrary to tradition, the evidence shows that pancreatic enzymes including trypsin, lipase, and amylase survive the duodenal environment largely intact and active. In a 1975 study, Legg and Spencer reported their experiences with the three enzymes stored for four weeks in alkaline human duodenal juice at various temperatures.[101] All three seemed fairly stable kept at –20°C, with 85% of the trypsin retained in its active state. At 5°C, 70% of the trypsin remained potent. At room temperature, losses were more substantial, though even after 4 days, 70% of trypsin remained viable, a rather substantial amount. Clearly, pancreatic enzymes appear stable in duodenal juices, even at room temperature, even for a considerable period of time.

Contemporary critics have long proclaimed the third obstacle, the improbable absorption of pancreatic enzymes through the intestinal mucosa, as the most daunting, in their minds precluding any systemic benefit from orally ingested preparations. In the standard teaching, with each meal the pancreas must pour out a substantial quantity of newly minted enzymes, which will gradually digest themselves away along with the food. This scenario requires that the gland must continually synthesize enormous amounts of all enzymes in constant preparation for the next meal, 24 hours a day, for the lifetime of the organism.[102]

Yet again, the actual scientific data contradicts cherished traditions. Over the past three decades, the physiologists Charles Liebow, currently at the State University of New York at Buffalo, and who taught at Cornell Medical College during my days there, and Stephen Rothman, of the University of California, San Francisco, have investigated the absorption of activated pancreatic enzymes as well as their precursors.

In their long years of research, these two investigators focused on the recycling of pancreatic enzymes secreted into the intestinal tract during digestion. As their first premise, they thought it impossible that the pancreas could create the copious enzyme supply needed for each meal de novo as experts have long assumed. In a series of elegant experiments they demonstrated that contrary to accepted dogma, the enzyme load secreted by the pancreas during meals isn't destroyed, but instead largely reabsorbed and recycled, in what they refer to as an "enteropancreatic" process, akin to the enterohepatic recirculation of bile salts.

In an early article on the subject entitled "Enteropancreatic Circulation of Digestive Enzymes," published in *Science* in 1975, Liebow and Rothman reported on the absorption of enzymes both in laboratory models as well as in live animals. They conclude that the enzymes easily pass through the intestinal mucosa:

> Digestive enzyme in the blood can be derived from at least two sources—the acinar cell itself and from the intestinal lumen via the bloodstream. The intestinal epithelium is permeable to a variety of proteins; for digestive enzymes in particular, substantial elastase, chymotrypsin, and trypsin permeabilities have been reported. We examined chymotrypsinogen permeability by comparing the mucosal to serosal flux of [$^3$H]chymotrypsinogen relative to that for [$^{131}$I]albumin across gut sacs prepared from rabbit ileum . . . nevertheless, we found that the permeability of the ileal membrane to chymotrypsinogen expressed per unit of concentration gradient was some nine times greater than that found for albumin . . .
>
> The existence of an enteropancreatic circulation for at least some digestive enzymes seems clear.[103]

Not surprisingly, their initial findings met with strong resistance from fellow physiologists, who despite the formidable evidence relentlessly stuck to the old belief that pancreatic enzymes cannot be absorbed through the intestinal lining. To their credit, Liebow and Rothman continued their studies, eventually summarizing their experience as well as the controversy still lingering over their findings in a lengthy review article entitled "Conservation of Digestive Enzymes" appearing in the January 2002 issue of *Physiology Reviews*. Their article begins:

> In this review we summarize experiments whose implications were of great interest when they were first reported. They pro-

vided unexpected evidence that the conventional belief that every meal is digested by an entirely new complement of digestive enzymes is incorrect. The data suggested that instead of being completely degraded in the small bowel with the food they digest, a large fraction of the digestive enzymes secreted by the pancreas are absorbed and recycled in an enteropancreatic circulation.[102]

The authors then proceed to catalogue in some detail the results of their experiments over the years, before essentially demolishing their critics. After some 16 pages, they conclude:

> As we reexamined the evidence for a conservation of digestive enzymes, we found it no less compelling than we did 25 years ago. Likewise, we found the studies that question its existence as incomplete as they seemed to us all those years ago . . .

> The traditional single pass view of digestion in which a completely new complement of digestive enzymes is manufactured for each meal has the curious consequence of requiring the organism to be particularly wasteful in its expenditure of energy to manufacture these costly molecules to meet its needs for sustenance . . . when just the opposite would seem desirable.[102]

Liebow and Rothman show that pancreatic enzymes present in the small intestine don't self-destruct, but survive to be largely and efficiently assimilated into the bloodstream for reuse. Though the two researchers have specifically studied the fate of enzymes secreted into the duodenum by the pancreas, the same rule presumably holds true for enzymes provided in supplement form.

To summarize, orally ingested pancreatic enzymes may easily survive the alleged ravages of hydrochloric acid in the stomach, the alkaline environment of the duodenum, and can then pass into the systemic circulation, with little loss along the way. The scientific documentation as reported in the literature therefore suggests that oral preparations can have a systemic effect.

# CHAPTER 11

# The Stability of Oral Enzyme Preparations

In the US, many pharmaceutical companies market enzyme products meant for oral consumption, either as prescription items for treatment of pancreatic insufficiency, or over the counter as digestive aids. Nearly all pancreatic enzyme preparations, including 36 prescription varieties, have been manufactured according to the Levin method or some variation thereof, involving the extraction of nearly all fat with simultaneous activation of most if not all proenzymes. Viokase, the traditional Viobin brand now owned by a separate company, contains less than 1% fat in the tablet and has a high degree of proteolytic activity, according to the specifications for the product.

Over the years, we have nonetheless continued recommending our minimally processed, unpurified formulation, with most of the enzymes in the precursor form and with much of the fat left intact. We believe this product suits our needs best, and have resisted changing the preparation.

In assessing the value of any enzyme product, we must consider its stability and its efficacy. In terms of the first issue, we believe our product to be quite stable over time; several years ago our manufacturer tested a batch from some five years earlier, which appeared to be as active as when initially encapsulated. On the other hand, we have long suspected, based on the literature, that enzymes processed according to the Levin methodology, with the enzyme component highly active and the fat removed, might be less stable. Evidence both old and new supports this supposition.

In a 1993 report entitled "Comparative In Vitro and In Vivo Studies of Enteric-Coated Pancrelipase Preparations for Pancreatic Insufficiency," the authors Thomson et al tested different enzyme products for stability and clinical effect. They describe significant losses in potency over time, as well as great variation in actual activity in different batches of the same brand name preparation:

> . . . the variation in enzyme activity between different batches of the same preparations related to time since manufacture and the decline of activity (especially lipase and amylase which showed an approximate decrease of 15–20% over an 8-month period) of a batch with time, which is not widely appreciated, may stimulate the clinician to objectively assess absorption following prescription of the same preparation with a different batch number or the same batch number after a prolonged storage time—even though it may still be within the expiry date quoted by the manufacturers.[104]

More recent evidence confirms that many if not the majority of enzyme products available by prescription provide erratic levels of enzyme activity, rarely what the label might claim. The problem came to a head in April 2004, when the FDA issued a notice that all manufacturers of prescription enzymes used in the treatment of pancreatic insufficiency must, within four years, provide evidence of stability and efficacy or else remove their product from the marketplace.

According to official documents published from that time, the FDA had received numerous complaints from physicians prescribing enzymes for pancreatic insufficiency. Apparently, clinical results could vary enormously from brand to brand and even with different bottles of the same brand. In response, the FDA conducted its own evaluation of available prescription enzymes, which revealed great discrepancy between their assessment of potency and what the label might claim.

A "Question and Answers" statement posted on the FDA website April 27, 2004, discusses the FDA's findings and new regulations for manufacturers. The article summarizes the problem as follows:

> Over the years, FDA has received reports of problems associated with these drugs [pancreatic enzymes]. Initially, the reports dealt with adverse events associated with high doses of enzymes leading to strictures of the intestines (narrowing of the digestive tract). More recently the Agency has received a number of reports claiming that these drug products do not have the expected therapeutic effect. There are many reasons why certain products may be subtherapeutic, including inactive ingredients or inadequate amounts of active drug in the capsule.[105]

Note that in the above, the FDA document mentions evidence of intestinal strictures occurring in certain patients ingesting large doses of pancreatic enzymes. This statement refers specifically to reports of fibrosing colonopathy observed in children with cystic fibrosis prescribed a particular form of pancreatic enzymes. Researchers in England first described the syndrome in 1994, three years after a "microencapsulated" high potency enzyme product first became available in the US and Europe.[106] In response to the initial cases reported in the literature, manufacturers voluntarily withdrew this formulation from the marketplace. In more recent years, we have seen no reports indicating a continuing problem.

The syndrome seemed to have been restricted to children with cystic fibrosis using the microencapsulated form, since it had never been described prior to 1991. In my experience over the past 27 years, first evaluating thousands of Kelley patients and more recently in our own practice, we have never seen this problem.

A press release dated April 27, 2004 reports the concerns of the Acting FDA Commissioner, Dr. Lester M. Crawford, about the problems with prescription enzymes:

> Variations in the potency of pancreatic extract drug product are unacceptable. Patients with exocrine pancreatic insufficiency disorders rely on these drugs to provide the enzymes they need to digest food properly. If the label contains an inaccurate

statement about a particular product's potency, then the patient
is at risk for receiving too much or too little of the medicine,"
said Dr. Lester M. Crawford . . . [107]

Clearly, the stability of enzyme preparations, most manufactured according to the Levin method, remains a serious and ongoing issue requiring recent FDA intervention. We can offer our own explanations of why these products might deteriorate significantly, even under routine storage conditions.

There are two factors to consider, the high level of activated proteases present, coupled with the minimal amounts of fat. Instinctively one might think a highly active material might be susceptible to auto-digestion sitting on the shelf at room temperature. After all, enzymes are themselves proteins, so when packed together in their activated form, they can begin attacking one another, converting the mixture into inactive peptides and amino acids. One might also assume that a capsule consisting largely of inactive precursors might be more resistant to such suicidal deterioration.

Though we believe the auto-digestion of activated enzymes does contribute to the instability of commercial brands, this process itself might be set off by the near absence of fat. The literature does provide clues suggesting that highly activated preparations with the "inert" fat extracted might deteriorate under normal storage conditions, while ours, consisting of largely precursors with the fat intact, might more effectively resist degradation. In a paper published in 1982, Muller and Ghale of the Institute of Child Health, London, reported one of the most thorough investigations of pancreatic enzyme stability under normal physiological conditions.[108] Though these scientists were primarily concerned with the fate of enzymes in the duodenum, their findings help explain why purified, highly active pancreatin tablets or capsules in a bottle might lose potency over time.

In their ingenious series of studies, Muller and Ghale evaluated the stability of enzymes secreted by the pancreas into duodenal juice. In a first set of experiments, the investigators assessed enzyme potency after consumption of a standardized Lundh test meal, often used to assess pancreatic function. The Lundh formula, usually administered by a tube inserted through the abdominal wall into the duodenum, consists of 5% protein, 6% fat, and 15% carbohydrate.

In the initial experiments, the researchers extracted the duodenal juice, which they then stored at a temperature of –20°C for up to a year. In the second experiment, duodenal fluids were collected in the absence of food but after injection of cholecystokinin or secretin, two hormones that stimulate the secretion of pancreatic enzymes into the small intestine. Once again, the juice was stored at –20°C for up to a year.

Normally, purified trypsin in solution begins auto-digestion even at temperatures as low as –70°C.[108] However, Muller and Ghale found that the enzymes secreted in the presence of a meal retained near-total potency at one year at –20°C, whereas those released in response to hormonal stimulus with no food present rapidly deteriorated. The authors proposed that in the absence of food, whether protein, fat, or carbohydrate, the auto-digestion cascade begins fairly quickly whereas the presence of food retards the process quite impressively. These studies suggest that pancreatic enzymes including trypsin do not deteriorate during the digestive process, if food is present:

> It was concluded from these studies that juices collected after a test meal stimulus can be stored for prolonged periods of time at –20°C without significant loss of enzyme activity. In hormonally stimulated juices, amylase is more stable than lipase or trypsin . . . [108]

Muller and Ghale suggest that the food components of the test meal themselves served as stabilizing factors for the various classes of enzymes:

> Theoretically, the observed differences in stability of lipase and trypsin could have resulted from a stabilising factor in the test meal itself or from the *in-vivo* production of either a stabilising factor after pancreatic stimulation by a test meal or a labilising factor after stimulation by exogenous hormones. The possibility that there was a stabilising factor in the test meal was stud-

ied by *in-vitro* addition experiments which showed that the test meal, its individual constituents, and glycerol could all stabilise lipase and trypsin activities for at least *one month*[Italics ours].[108]

Muller and Ghale report specifically that corn oil—a pure lipid—nicely protected against degradation.

We believe that the high percentage of precursors in our product helps prevent deterioration during normal storage. But based on the Muller experiments, we suspect that the non-enzymatic components of our largely unpurified pancreatin, especially the substantial quantity of fat, more than 10 times the amount in most products, also protect the enzymes from self-annihilation. In contrast, we think the high levels of initial enzyme activity coupled with the lack of fat in most if not all commercial preparations might contribute to the instability reported in the literature.

Earlier, we mentioned the work of Regan et al, Graham et al, and Dutta et al, all of whom blamed the lack of clinical efficacy noted for various enzyme formulations on acid denaturation in the stomach.[96-98] We believe these researchers blamed an innocent bystander; based on the evidence, even before these products had been consumed, most likely considerable activity had already been lost.

# CHAPTER 12

# Active Enzyme Versus Precursor: Which Works Best Against Cancer?

Ezra Levin developed his processing method convinced that the best pancreatic enzyme, for both pharmaceutical and industrial use, would contain minimal fat, and provide most if not all enzymes in the active configuration.[87] Kelley followed suit, believing, apparently to his grave, that the more purified of "useless" fat and the more active the product, the better. Kelley was actually quite familiar with the Ezra Levin patent, which he treated like his own personal enzyme Bible and which he quoted often, to help justify his belief that more active means better.

During the mid to late 1990s, we learned that Dr. Kelley—who had been travelling the country to avoid imagined enemies of his therapy—had begun seeing patients again, prescribing his latest enzyme concoction that he claimed was the strongest and the best. One of his supporters actually sent me a copy of a laboratory analysis of the supplement describing a "29X" potency, higher than we had thought possible. The lab report indicated the presence of large amounts of pure trypsin and chymotrypsin, apparently added for extra effect. Though we certainly don't know the details, we also heard through the alternative grapevine that few patients who followed this newest incarnation of his treatment did well.

We have no doubt that our preparation, consisting of mostly precursors with a modest level of enzymes in the active form, with all the various pancreatic tissue components intact including the fat, retains potency over time under the usual conditions of supplement storage at room temperature. We have also long believed that the high percentage of precursors in the preparation not only lends added stability, but might actually provide a far more powerful anti-cancer punch.

Though the French physician Lucien Corvisart first described trypsin in 1856, when Beard pursued his investigations 50 years later scientists still knew little about the dynamics of pancreatic enzymes, their secretion in a precursor form, or their subsequent activation in the small intestine by mucosal enterokinase.[109] Only years after Beard's death would physiologists discover the intricacies of pancreatic enzyme physiology. Since Beard apparently knew nothing of proenzymes, he could only assume that active trypsin provided the anti-cancer effect he had observed in his laboratory and clinical studies.

But as Novak and Trnka argue in their excellent article "Proenzyme Therapy of Cancer," the formulations Beard recommended for treatment unbeknownst to him most likely provided a high percentage of precursors.[109] The authors point out that Beard always insisted that for best results, the pancreatin must be prepared from fresh animal glands quickly processed—material which would provide most of the enzymes in their inactive conformation. Though Beard always identified trypsin as the primary anti-cancer enzyme, Novak and Trnka insist the proenzymes such as trypsinogen and not the active configurations provided benefit in Beard's investigations.

In their own animal and human studies, Novak and Trnka discovered that a pancreatin consisting mostly of precursors and not active enzymes worked best against cancer.[109] Active pancreatic proteases present in the systemic circulation, as a start, appear susceptible to neutralization by a series of enzyme-blocking molecules called serpins present in blood. On the other hand, the proenzymes seem completely immune to such assault. Subsequently, at the cancer cell membrane—but not in normal tissues—the precursors quickly convert into their active conformation capable of attacking the malignant tissue directly and effectively. As they write in their "Abstract":

> We hypothesize that the provision of zymogens [proenzymes], rather than the enzymes, was of crucial importance to the clini-

cal effectiveness in the human trials conducted by Beard and his co-workers. The precursor nature of the active enzymes may offer protection against numerous serpins present in the tissues and blood. Experimental evidence supports the assertion that the conversion from proenzyme to enzyme occurs selectively on the surface of the tumor cells, but not on normal cells. We believe that this selectivity of activation is responsible for the antitumor/antimetastatic effect of proenzyme therapy and low toxicity to normal cells or tumor host. . . These findings support the conclusion that proteolysis is the active mechanism of the proenzyme treatment.[109]

Though Novak and Trnka used only injectable enzymes in their studies, we believe the same rule applies to our orally ingested, largely unpurified, predominantly precursor product. We suspect a high percentage of the proenzymes do not undergo activation in their journey through the stomach and duodenum, but remain in their inactive form to be absorbed as such. Then, after circulating unaffected by the various enzyme blockers in the blood, at the cancer cell membrane the precursors unleash a potent anti-cancer effect.

But can these proenzymes really make their way through the intestinal mucosa as efficiently as the somewhat smaller, active enzymes? Indeed, they can, as Liebow and Rothman argue. First, the pair report that not all precursor enzymes secreted by the pancreas during a meal activate in the alkaline duodenum. Instead, they have documented that many remain in the proenzyme form to be taken up into the systemic circulation.[102] We suspect that in a similar way, most of the proenzymes in our preparation are absorbed unchanged.

The research of Novak and Trnka also helps explain why Dr. Kelley's successes fell off considerably when he switched to a product consisting of mostly activated enzymes. Not only was this defatted preparation we believe unstable on the shelf, but its complement of enzymes would have been in the wrong form in any event for optimal anti-cancer effect.

Finally, we would like to make one additional point about the fat content in our product. As discussed, we assume the lipid present serves as a stabilizing factor to prevent auto-digestion.[108] We also believe, today more strongly than 20 years ago, that the fat fraction Levin saw as worthless filler provides considerable biological activity that may work cooperatively with the proteolytic component. As researchers unraveled the mysteries of fat during the 1990s, the evidence showed it to be not just an inert collection of stored energy, but a very active endocrine organ involved in many physiological activities. In a 2006 review of the subject entitled "Adipose Tissue-Derived Factors: Impact on Health and Disease," Trujillo and Scherer summarize in detail the newly emerging field of fat endocrinology:

> Studies in the late 1980s have demonstrated that adipocytes can secrete a number of factors and that the secretion of some of these factors is affected by metabolic dysregulation. However, the concept describing the adipocyte as an endocrine cell did not gain general acceptance until several additional factors were identified in which expression was highly enriched in adipocytes, such as leptin and Acrp30/adiponectin. For the past 10 yr, endocrine aspects of adipose tissue function have become an extremely active area of research, and several additional hormones have been discovered. Generally, these adipose tissue-derived factors are referred to as adipokines. These adipokines influence a number of important systemic phenomena and interact in the process with a large number of different organ systems.[110]

Researchers currently recognize two forms of storage fat, brown and white adipose tissue. The brown form specifically helps provide heat energy when needed as the external temperature drops. White adipose tissue synthesizes a series of hormones and cytokines, including, to name but a few, adiponectin, which increases insulin sensitivity and protects against heart disease; aromatase, which efficiently converts circulating testosterone into estradiol; angiotensin, which constricts blood vessels and raises blood pressure; and interleukin-6 and tumor necrosis factor, both pro-inflammatory cytokines. We suspect that many other hormones, cytokines and growth factors, still unknown, remain to be discovered specifically in the fat of the pancreas gland, molecules that very well may enhance the anti-cancer activity of the enzymes.

So in summary, the evidence supports that an unpurified pancreatic preparation with substantial fat, providing a mixture of some active enzymes but mostly precursors, remains more stable on the shelf than a highly purified, highly activated formulation. After ingestion, pancreatic enzymes, both active and in precursor form, survive hydrochloric acid assault in the stomach, and the alkaline environment of the duodenum. Both active and precursor enzymes can then be absorbed through the intestinal mucosa into the systemic circulation. Based on the work of Novak and Trnka, the proenzymes provided by our product would be immune to the anti-enzyme serpins circulating in the blood, then activate at the tumor site where they are most needed.

# Conclusion to Part II

So as we close Part II, we want to give Dr. Beard credit for his efforts to unravel one of the great mysteries of mammalian embryology, the transformation of the trophoblast from an undifferentiated, proliferative, highly invasive, migratory, and angiogenic tissue into the differentiated and non-aggressive mature placenta. Beard determined that the trophoblast begins this change in earnest at about week 8 after conception in humans, at the same time, he proposed, that the embryonic pancreas first becomes active. Though he might not have been completely correct in all the minute details—for example, he could not have known that fetal liver production of trypsin and other proteolytic enzymes might exceed that of the early pancreas—his assumption that the trophoblast begins changing character in the presence of these enzymes appears to have been well founded.

Beard furthermore insisted that cancer arose only from misplaced trophoblast growing from a vagrant germ cell, stirred into replicative activity—a view contemporary evidence to some extent supports. Consequently, his leap of faith, his suggestion that if pancreatic proteolytic enzymes ultimately regulate trophoblast development, they should equally as efficiently control malignancy seems, from the vantage point of 2008, reasonable. Certainly, both past and present laboratory and clinical evidence, including our own experience over the past 25 years, does in our opinion confirm his belief that the pancreatic proteolytic enzymes—not our immune or any other system—represent the body's main defense against cancer and the most effective tool against the disease once it takes hold. Though again he may not have been always accurate in the finer points—Beard couldn't know for example that his most effective enzyme preparation probably provided far more precursor than active protease—in his elegant research of long ago he may have uncovered not only the mechanism for the life-sustaining transformation of the early trophoblast, but the solution for the life-destroying disease of cancer.

# My Review of Dr. Kelley

*(By Dr. Gonzalez)*

As discussed earlier, during the 1960s the eccentric dentist Dr. William Kelley developed his own variation of enzyme treatment, relying on orally ingested preparations. In addition to large doses of pancreatic enzymes, Kelley's program included individualized diets and supplement protocols, as well as detoxification routines such as the coffee enemas. Dr. Kelley came to fame at a time of great repression organized against alternative medicine in general, and particularly against anyone suggesting a nutritional treatment might have benefit against advanced cancer. Kelley was at particular risk because as a dentist, he lacked the legal right to treat cancer in the first place. He was repeatedly attacked in the press, vilified as a "quack," and investigated by numerous government agencies. He was thrown in jail as a public menace, had his dental license revoked for five years for practicing medicine, spent his earnings defending himself against government assaults and saw his family life fall apart. But he, like Beard, never relented, and survived because his successes created an extraordinary word-of-mouth network that brought an endless stream of patients to his Grapevine, Texas, and later his Winthrop, Washington offices.

I met Dr. Kelley by chance in 1981 during the summer following my second year of medical school. At that time, he seemed completely modest and unassuming, seeking only to have his work properly evaluated so that if the approach had merit, it might become more widely accessible to patients in need. I was fortunate to have as a mentor at Cornell

University Medical College the late Robert A Good, M.D., Ph.D., at the time Director of Sloan-Kettering, who encouraged a review of Kelley's cases. I couldn't have asked for a better guide than Dr. Good, the most published author in the history of medicine, the man *The New York Times* described as the "Founder of Modern Immunology." Among his many accomplishments, he helped decipher the important role of the thymus, and performed the first bone marrow transplant in history.

Under Dr. Good's direction, I began a student project evaluating Dr. Kelley's methods, his patients, his successes and failures. Dr. Good encouraged me in my efforts, telling me that even if Kelley proved to be a fraud, I would learn much medicine from a project of my own choosing, developed out of my own enthusiasm.

Despite the eccentricities in Kelley's behavior that would only worsen until his death in 2005, I quickly found evidence of patient after patient with appropriately diagnosed, biopsy proven advanced cancer, who were alive five, even 10 years since first beginning the enzyme therapy. What began as a mere student investigation evolved into a full-fledged research project, completed while I was an immunology fellow under Dr. Good at All Children's Hospital in Florida, where, after leaving Sloan, he had moved to establish a bone marrow transplant unit.

I eventually interviewed and evaluated over 1000 of Kelley's patients, concentrating on a group of 455 who seemed to have done well under his care. From this population, I wrote up in detail 50 case reports, representing 26 different types of cancer, for each documenting outcomes in terms of disease regression and survival far beyond what would normally be expected by the standards of conventional oncology. Even today, 20 years later, when I review my efforts I am still impressed by Kelley's achievement.

By 1986, I had put the results of my five-year investigation into monograph form, which I then hoped to publish. To my disappointment and surprise, despite my careful labors and serious intent, I could not get the book published either in its entirety as a monograph, or as a summary journal article. The responses from editors ran the gamut from disbelief and accusations of fraud, to fear that the book would generate so much controversy their publishing careers might be ruined. No editor, even those who accepted the data as real, had the courage to take on the project.

Our failure to publish the study had a very damaging effect on Dr. Kelley. It appeared to him that all doors had closed, that his work would never be accepted for what he believed it was, a promising answer to a deadly disease. In 1986, he closed down his office and eventually disappeared from sight. After 1987 I never spoke to him again.

Over the years, particularly with the rise of the Internet, a number of myths have sprouted about my study, usually originating from those who have never read it. I have even heard the claim made that the study had no value because the patients didn't really have cancer.

Indeed, the 50 patients described had been diagnosed with cancer by conventional physicians, and Dr. Good himself approved all for inclusion in the monograph. Though widely known as a pioneering immunologist, prior to assuming the Directorship at Sloan-Kettering, Dr. Good had served as Head of the Department of Pathology at the University of Minnesota, and was a renowned cancer pathologist. He and I together evaluated each and every case that ultimately made its way into the monograph, in many instances reviewing the actual pathology slides together.

Two of the 50 lacked confirmatory biopsies, but due to the remarkable nature of each patient history, Dr. Good suggested I include both in my final report. In the first case, at the time of diagnosis the patient had collapsed into the terminal phases of unresectable biliary duct malignancy, with obvious liver failure. He did undergo exploratory surgery, with the intent of relieving a bile duct obstructed by tumor. However, the disease appeared so extensive the surgeon chose to end the operation without completing the proposed procedure. He even decided against performing a biopsy, which he feared might risk hemorrhage in an already unstable patient.

The operative note describes the findings clearly:

> Carcinoma of the right hepatic bile duct with extension into the left and common hepatic ducts with total obstruction . . .

Post surgery, the patient underwent a course of palliative radiation to help reduce the biliary blockage. After finishing the treatment, the patient subsequently learned of Kelley, pursued the regimen as best as he could and survived nearly six years after diagnosis before succumbing to liver failure, brought on by his original extensive disease.

In the second case, the patient underwent exploratory laparotomy after developing jaundice secondary to biliary obstruction. At surgery, he was found to have a large inoperable pancreatic mass with liver metastases. The surgeon performed a palliative bypass procedure, but did not biopsy any of the lesions because of the clearly terminal nature of the disease, and his fear the procedure might provoke severe hemorrhage.

The operative note states:

> On opening the abdominal cavity, immediately noted was a large nodular lesion occupying the head of the pancreas and extending and going downwards . . . Pancreatic body was also felt and was grossly enlarged and nodular and firm . . . the liver was smooth, there was evident metastatic spread.
>
> The mass itself, occupied most of the c-loop of the duodenum and the mass extending downward overlying the posterior mesenteric muscle . . .
>
> No attempt at pancreatic biopsy was deemed necessary because of the obvious findings and because of the dangers associated with this procedure . . .

Thereafter, the patient began the Kelley regimen and experienced a remarkable response, surviving 12 years with an excellent quality of life before dying of old age, with no sign of cancer at the time of his death.

In the remaining 48 cases, biopsy studies confirmed malignant disease. Many of the patients had been diagnosed at major institutions, including five at the Mayo clinic, four at Memorial Sloan-Kettering, three at Stanford, and one at M.D. Anderson.

# Four Kelley Patients

*(By Dr. Gonzalez)*

In this chapter, I include four representative patient histories from my original Kelley monograph entitled *One Man Alone,* completed in 1986 and then updated in mid-1987.[111] Note that I report survival information as of my last contact with the patient. I have also included references, as appropriate, as they appeared in the original monograph.

**PATIENT #7:** This patient underwent a right mastectomy in 1970 for what was thought to be localized breast cancer. After surgery, she received no additional treatment, and did well until 1973, when she developed a tumor in the left breast treated, like the first, with mastectomy. She again received no additional therapy, 1973 being long before the advent of aggressive adjuvant chemotherapy for breast cancer.

In mid-1974, Patient #7 developed pain along the length of the vertebral column extending into the right shoulder, associated with persistent fatigue and chronic depression. Her doctors initially suspected her symptoms were unrelated to her cancer, but when she worsened in the spring of 1975, she underwent a diagnostic work-up. X-ray studies revealed a lesion in the fifth lumbar segment of the spine, described as "indicative of osteolytic metastasis from the breast carcinoma." A bone scan confirmed multiple lesions consistent with metastatic disease in both the skull and right shoulder blade, reported as "focal abnormal uptakes of skull and tip of right scapula (shoulder), possibility of metastatic disease."

The patient then underwent palliative oophorectomy (removal of the ovaries), to reduce her estrogen load and hopefully slow the progression of her disease. Despite the surgery, Patient #7 was told she most probably would not live out the year. In desperation, she subsequently decided to investigate alternative cancer therapies, learned of Dr. Kelley and began the nutritional program in the summer of 1975.

Within six months, the persistent pain, fatigue and depression resolved. A bone scan performed at the end of 1975 showed some improvement, and a third bone scan, from mid-1976, indicated complete resolution of disease. When last contacted in 1987, she was alive and well with no evidence of cancer, 12 years out from her recurrence.

In this case, though oophorectomy was known to improve pain and at times lead to tumor regression if only briefly, the procedure was strictly palliative and does not cure metastatic breast cancer. My monograph states:

> As discussed previously, the five-year survival rate for patients with metastatic breast cancer approaches 0.0%, regardless of conventional therapy administered. And oophorectomy, which may lead to symptomatic improvement in this group, does not cure metastatic breast cancer. Hellman reports overall response rates for the procedure, in those women with estrogen dependent disease, in the range of 30–40%. However, even among these patients, the benefit lasts only nine to 12 months on average, with little survival advantage.[112(p945)]

> In summary, this patient developed evidence of metastases after successive mastectomies for recurring breast carcinoma. Although she did undergo oophorectomy, Patient #7 continued to deteriorate after the procedure. She received neither chemotherapy nor radiation, and her extensive disease and many symptoms resolved only after she began the Kelley program.

Even today, with all the innovative drugs that have been developed since I completed my Kelley project, metastatic breast cancer remains incur-

able. This patient's extraordinary disease-free survival can only be attributed to the Kelley regimen.

**PATIENT #8:** In mid-1977, this patient experienced episodic vaginal
bleeding that gradually worsened over a six-month period. After biopsy
of a cervical mass in January 1978 revealed "invasive squamous cell carcinoma of the cervix," Patient #8 was referred to the W.W. Cross Cancer
Institute in Edmonton, Alberta. There, the diagnosis was confirmed and
the patient staged with early 1B disease. At that point, her physicians
recommended radiation therapy, beginning with a two-step regimen of
radium insertions into the cervical area followed by 3500 rads of external beam radiation to the pelvis. The doctors hoped that if the tumor
shrunk sufficiently they could then proceed with surgery. However,
Patient #8, already knowledgeable about alternative cancer therapies,
suggested to her physicians a nutritional approach. In my monograph I
describe the response as appearing in the official record:

> "Apparently she (Mrs. ——) is a little worried about radiation
> therapy treatment," wrote her physician in his notes, "but we
> have tried to explain to her the only orthodox treatments at the
> present time for her condition are surgical or radiotherapeutic
> and that in view of the surgical complication rates, it is our policy
> in this clinic . . . to employ radiation as a routine. . . . I think both
> she and her daughter are a little doubtful about accepting this and
> she wonders whether some dietary methods may be helpful. I
> have informed her that there is no evidence known to me to sug-
> gest that diet will influence cancer to any significant degree and
> that any delay in commencing treatment will almost certainly
> lead to impaired chances of cure . . . "

After some delay, she eventually completed the insertion therapy but decided to discontinue external beam radiation after completing only
1150 rads to the anterior and posterior pelvis over a five day period.
Her doctor was not pleased:

> "I had a long talk with her and daughter [sic], the patient is obvi-
> ously got [sic] an Ostrich syndrome," her physician wrote in an

> April 14, 1978 note. "She thinks that if she doesn't have any
> treatment the disease will go away . . . . I have emphasized that her
> maximum chances of cure and control of her disease are a full
> treatment now and that we cannot add on in the future to the
> partial treatment she has taken to date."

Patient #8 nonetheless declined further conventional treatment, and for
a time pursued no therapy of any type. By late April 1978, she began to
deteriorate rapidly, describing, when I interviewed her years later, severe
weakness, fatigue, and recurrent vaginal bleeding. She returned to
Cross, where a cervical smear confirmed recurrent cancer. Despite the
diagnosis, she once again refused to resume radiation, instead choosing
to consult with Dr. Kelley. However, she did not begin her prescribed nutritional regimen, she told me, because of her family's opposition to any
alternative approach.

Throughout the summer of 1978, the cancer grew unchecked. In
September 1978, after she developed a partial urinary tract obstruction
caused by enlarging pelvic tumors, a renogram confirmed declining
function in both kidneys. Patient #8 still refused all orthodox intervention and in late October 1978, after her vaginal bleeding worsened,
Patient #8 was admitted on an emergency basis to Misericordia
Hospital. Her doctors noted on exam a large abdominal mass extending
into the bladder as reported in the records.

> The lower abdomen was tender and it was felt likely that there was
> some urinary retention. However because of the tumor mass rising
> out of the pelvis, it was difficult to assess . . .

After blood tests showed her to be severely anemic with a hemoglobin of
7.4 g/dL (normal 12–16), she required multiple transfusions before finally stabilizing. Subsequently, an oncologist called in to evaluate the
situation recommended no treatment other than pain control, believing
her to be terminal. She then began the Brompton Cocktail, a highly potent pain mixture usually reserved for dying cancer patients. Family
members, whom I interviewed, were told the patient most probably
would not live more than several weeks and at their suggestion, she was

discharged from the hospital on November 3, 1978, so she might die at home. On the official summary from that date, the provisional diagnosis reads "CA UTERUS—TERMINAL" with a secondary diagnosis of "METASTATIC SPREAD TO ABDOMINAL CAVITY."

The records also discuss the opinion of the consulting oncologist:

> The patient was seen by Dr. —— in consultation and he noted the marked anemia and the frozen pelvis with carcinoma. He felt that he was unable to examine her adequately rectally because of the hemorrhoids and he agreed that she should continue with Foley catheter drainage (continuous) and other supportive measures.
>
> Initially he felt that chemotherapy might be considered but subsequently he decided not to. She was also seen by Social Services in consultation and they arranged for VON [visiting nurse] and homemaker to go into the house.

After her discharge from Misericordia, Patient #8 was readmitted the following day, at which time the large tumor in her abdomen was again noted:

> Abdomen showed marked tenderness with a hard tumor mass rising up out the pelvis.

The family planned to place her in hospice care, but at that point Patient #8 contacted Dr. Kelley, who suggested she start the full program at once. Because of his support, she insisted on returning home during the second week of November 1978, so she might begin her protocol. This time around, Patient #8 stuck religiously to the prescribed regimen, and quickly improved. Over the following year, her abdominal tumors regressed completely by her own accounting, her kidney function returned to normal, and she was able to discontinue all pain medications without experiencing narcotic withdrawal. At the time we last spoke in 1987, she was in excellent health, apparently cancer-free, still taking pancreatic enzymes, more than nine years out from her terminal prognosis. She reported a recent Pap smear and abdominal ultrasound were both negative for malignancy. She regretted that she didn't refuse all radiation and begin the Kelley program sooner, thinking her course would have been much easier had she followed her instincts.

This case does not require much analysis. A 1978 biopsy confirmed recurrent cervical cancer after a course of radiation implants. Initially, as Patient #8 pursued no treatment, the disease progressed quickly to a terminal stage, as documented in the medical records. With hospice her only other option, she began the Kelley program in earnest with subsequent total regression of her disease. Her long-term, nine-year disease-free survival can only be attributed to Kelley's therapy.

**PATIENT #17:** In April 1977 after developing a scrotal abscess and significant anemia requiring transfusion, Patient #17 was diagnosed at the Ochsner Clinic in New Orleans with acute myelocytic leukemia, confirmed by bone marrow biopsy. The oncologists at Ochsner, after warning the patient and his family that this malignancy represented the most aggressive form of leukemia, recommended he immediately begin treatment with the chemotherapy drugs thioguanine and cytosine arabinoside. Even with treatment, Patient #17 was told he most likely would not live a year.

Patient #17 reacted badly to the regimen, lapsing into severe congestive heart failure during the first cycle of therapy. After stabilizing, he received a second round of chemotherapy but subsequent bone marrow studies indicated he had failed to achieve remission, as documented in his oncologist's notes.

When after a third cycle of drugs the disease remained active, Patient #17 refused further treatment, began considering alternative approaches and decided to consult with Dr. Kelley in December 1977. At the time, he was quite ill, with severe fatigue and malaise. Thereafter, he followed the Kelley regimen faithfully, with gradual improvement in his symptoms to the point he returned to work full-time, while continuing the Kelley regimen. Subsequently, a bone marrow biopsy from July 1978, after he had completed eight months of his nutritional treatment, confirmed the disease finally to be in remission.

During the years of my study, I came to know this patient and his family quite well. Always diligent with his program, he remained a strong supporter of Dr. Kelley. He did eventually pass away in September 1984 from causes unrelated to his malignant disease, more than seven years after his terminal prognosis. He was thought to be completely cancer-free at the time of his death.

Acute myelocytic leukemia, even today, is one of the most deadly, aggressive cancers. Even with current chemotherapy regimens in 2009, only 10–15% of patient live five years. And though the regimen offered Patient #17 in 1977 might extend life, it was never considered curative.

My monograph states:

> The survival statistics for acute myelocytic leukemia remain abysmal, with the literature reporting an average lifespan for untreated patients diagnosed with the disease of only three months.[113(p807)] Even with aggressive therapy, only 10–15% of patients—at most—live five years, with survival rates declining considerably with increasing age.
>
> In adults with AML, prolonged survival, as rare as it is in any case, has been documented only with chemotherapy regimens that incorporate the drug daunorubicin, never given Patient #17.[112(p1422)] In a group of leukemic patients followed since 1967, five-year survival rate for patients receiving only cytosine arabinoside and thioguanine approaches 0%.[112(p1422)]
>
> After searching through the medical literature, I could find no evidence for an adult patient surviving five years on the drug regimen administered Patient #17. I decided to write an authority in the field of acute leukemias, Dr. Peter Wiernik, currently head of the Department of Oncology at the Albert Einstein College of Medicine, to ask if he knew of any such patients. Dr. Wiernik kindly responded:
>
> > I do not know of any five year or longer survivors of acute granulocytic [myelocytic] leukemia treated only with cytosine arabinoside and 6-thioguanine . . .
>
> It seems only reasonable, therefore, to attribute Patient #17's long-term survival to the Kelley program.

Furthermore, this patient, who completed only three cycles of a proposed lengthy course of treatment, achieved remission only after beginning the Kelley regimen. It seems reasonable today, as it did 20 years ago, to attribute his survival to his nutritional therapy.

**PATIENT #34:** In August 1982, during exploratory surgery for assumed gallbladder disease, this patient was found to have a tumor in the liver and an unresectable pancreatic mass. A biopsy of the liver lesion confirmed metastatic adenocarcinoma, most likely originating from a pancreatic primary.

A local oncologist who consulted with the patient told her no treatment could cure her disease and that she should get her "affairs in order." In the official records, the physician wrote: "The patient's prognosis is judged to be between 9 and 15 months at most."

In September 1982, Patient #34 decided to seek a second opinion at the Mayo Clinic where a CT scan revealed again an enlarged pancreas, and blood studies documented elevated liver function tests. Review of the biopsy slides confirmed the earlier diagnosis of metastatic pancreatic adenocarcinoma. At the conclusion of his consultation, the Mayo oncologist wrote, in the official discharge summary:

> I had a long discussion with her regarding treatment for her cancer. At the present time I would favor simply observation since we know of no known treatment that will necessarily prolong her life. Since she is feeling well at the present time I did not feel justified in making her symptomatic from the side effects of chemotherapy.

Once home, Patient #34 began investigating alternative cancer approaches and in December 1982 began the Kelley program. She later reported to me that within six months she returned to working 18 hours a day, seven days a week, running the family gas station. When she referred a patient to our office in the mid-1990s, she reported excellent health with no sign of cancer. I most recently heard from her in the spring of 2009, when she called to "check in." She reported feeling "great" except for some arthritis, and talked at length about her grand-children.

Since she refused follow-up radiographic studies after her initial diagnosis, I have no evidence of tumor regression, only her 27-year survival as of mid-2009. Certainly, for a disease that usually kills within 3–6 months, her long-term survival should itself prove treatment effect.

My discussion of pancreatic cancer statistics as appearing in the monograph reads as follows:

> Overall, pancreatic malignancies claimed 24,300 lives in 1987, making the disease the fourth most common cause of cancer-related death, and the incidence seems to be increasing yearly. Experts consider malignancy of the exocrine pancreas one of the deadliest of all neoplasms, with fewer than 2% of patients alive five years after diagnosis despite intensive treatment.[114(p652)]

My summary for this particular patient reads:

> Patient #34 responded very quickly to her protocol. Within six months, she was back to working 18 hours a day, seven days a week, running the family gas station, and today, nearly five years after her diagnosis, she is in excellent health. As she told me when I called her at her filling station, "I just don't have time to die."

# Our Recent Practice Experience With Enzyme Therapy

*(By Dr. Gonzalez)*

I n the fall of 1987, a year after finishing my research fellowship under Dr. Good, Dr. Isaacs and I returned to New York determined to keep the therapy alive. At that point, Dr. Good, having left Sloan, no longer had the power to help guide my treatment to the next level of clinical trials, so we agreed I would be best off seeing patients myself, and collecting my own data on the treatment approach, always with the hope of obtaining proper research support from the academic world. We parted friends.

In retrospect, 22 years later, I am somewhat amazed at how determined I was, and how sure that if I just kept trying, I would be able to win the battle, gain research backing, and ultimately prove the benefit of the treatment. Along the way, I made serious professional choices; once back in New York, a former professor of mine at Cornell who had remained in contact with me and who seemed to think I had some promise as an academic scientist, offered me a position in his group at Sloan-Kettering. But when he suggested I pursue more mainstream research projects instead of my flagrantly controversial work, I turned the offer down. Though touched by his interest and concern, I simply could not walk away from the enzyme treatment.

The work was initially very difficult since the patients who came to us invariably had very advanced disease. But we began having successes, victories that kept us going, patients who seemed to beat their cancer, many of whom are alive today. One such patient, the woman mentioned earlier with metastatic inflammatory breast cancer widely disseminated to the bone, today is alive and well more than 21 years since her original diagnosis, with scans long ago confirming total regression of disease. Another woman with aggressive breast cancer that had metastasized into the bone and liver came to me in 1990 after failing to respond to chemotherapy. She remains alive and well, 19 years from her terminal diagnosis. Then there is my patient with metastatic adenocarcinoma of the pancreas diagnosed in September 1991 with evidence of multiple cancerous lesions in the liver, in both adrenals, in the bone and lung. At last contact he had been alive some 15 years since first consulting me, with scans over the years showing total regression of his once widely metastatic disease.

In July 1993, the National Cancer Institute invited me to present case reports from my own practice, detailing patients with appropriately diagnosed poor prognosis cancer who had experienced tumor regression or unusual survival while following my therapy. Dr. Isaacs and I put together 25 cases for the session, attended by a large group of NCI scientists and lasting three hours. After the meeting, Dr. Michael Friedman, then Associate Director at the NCI, suggested we pursue as a next step a pilot study evaluating my approach in ten patients diagnosed with advanced adenocarcinoma of the pancreas. In such phase II clinical trials, as they are technically called, a promising new therapy is administered to patients with an aggressive cancer for which no effective standard treatment exists. A pilot study involves no control group, but can still give important information about a treatment. Since inoperable pancreatic cancer has such a grim prognosis, with an average survival in the range of 3–6 months, Dr. Friedman stated that if I could get three patients to live a year, he would consider that a significant success. From my experience with enzymes, I expected to do better.

We were fortunate to get funding for the study from Nestlé, the giant international food conglomerate. The then Vice President of the company in charge of research, Dr. Pierre Guesry, who had formerly been Medical Director of the Pasteur Institute in Paris, had learned of my work, became a supporter and convinced Nestlé to fund the study.

We finished the project and published the results in the June 1999 issue of the peer-reviewed research journal *Nutrition and Cancer*.[115] We eventually included 11 subjects, adding a patient when one dropped out. Of the 11, all had biopsy proven, inoperable disease, eight of the eleven had stage IV, and most had been very sick prior to consulting with us. All the patients were approved by a consulting oncologist and the late Dr. Ernst Wynder, one of the premier cancer epidemiologists of the 20th century. Of the eleven, nine lived more than one year, five lived more than two years, four lived more than three years, and two made it beyond four years, results far superior to any that had previously been reported for the disease. As a point of reference, in the clinical trial of Gemzar, a drug approved by the FDA for the treatment of pancreatic cancer in 1998, of 126 patients treated with chemotherapy not one lived longer than 19 months.[116] Yet this improvement in survival has been heralded as a "significant advance" over prior drug regimens.

In 1998, based on preliminary data from the pilot study, the NCI approved funding for a large scale, phase III clinical trial, testing our enzyme-nutritional approach in patients with advanced pancreatic cancer, but this time against a control group that would receive the best available chemotherapy. Eventually, the FDA approved the protocol and the National Center for Complementary and Alternative Medicine offered to put up the required funding. Columbia University, under the Chief of Oncology at the time and the Chief of Surgical Oncology, became the supervising institution in New York. Unfortunately, now years later, despite our earlier optimism the project remains unfinished, beset by bureaucratic difficulties, gross indifference and poor management by the Columbia and NCI team. That story I will tell in detail in another book.

As the NCI study bogged down, my friend Dr. Guesry at Nestlé provided funding for studies to test the enzyme treatment in animal models. A group at the Eppley Cancer Institute of the University of Nebraska, known for their investigations into the molecular biology of pancreatic cancer, agreed to take on the challenge. Dr. Parviz Pour, the supervisor of the animal work at Nebraska, has himself developed mouse models of pancreatic cancer that are used to test promising new treatments against the disease.

In May 2004, Dr. Pour published the results of the experiments in the peer reviewed journal *Pancreas* with Dr. Guesry and me listed as co-authors.[117] In these studies, the researchers evaluated the effect of our enzymes in nude mice injected with human pancreatic cancer cells of a particularly virulent strain. These animals lack a functional immune system, so normally transplanted or injected cancers grow very rapidly and kill quickly. In the first study, which measured survival, the mice were divided into two groups, one receiving our enzymes, the other given no therapy. The animals treated with our enzymes survived significantly longer than the untreated control group. Additionally, the enzyme mice appeared to be healthy, happy mice, even well into the study, in sharp contrast to the controls, who were listless, inactive, bloated, and obviously quite ill. Two of the mice in the treated group were doing so well they had to be sacrificed so the study could be brought to conclusion. We wonder how long they would have kept going.

In a second experiment, again the mice were divided into two groups, one administered our enzymes, the other untreated. This time, animals were periodically sacrificed and evaluated for tumor growth. The enzymes clearly reduced the proliferation of the tumors, which in the treated mice remained small and very localized. In the controls, tumors were considerably larger and more invasive.

We want to emphasize that the results are particularly significant because we had never used the enzymes to treat animals before, and decided to start at the dose per kilogram that we normally recommend for humans. Inbred laboratory mice metabolize most drugs far differently than we do, so that doses much higher than what would be given humans must be administered to achieve any effect. And, the experiments only evaluated the enzyme component of the treatment, not the additional vitamins, minerals, trace elements, and nutritious food we prescribe for our human patients. The animal chow also contained a fair amount of soy, which, however aggressively it may be pushed as a beneficial food, contains one of the most potent natural trypsin inhibitors known, the Bowman-Birk inhibitor.[118]

So we believe the results are important. As the authors wrote in the "Discussion" section, "In summary, PPE [Porcine Pancreatic Extracts] is the first experimentally and clinically proven agent for the effective treatment of PC [Pancreatic Cancer]. The significant advantages of PPE over any other currently available therapeutic modalities include its effects on physical condition, nutrition, and lack of toxicity."[117] Note that these results validate only the specific enzymes we use in our therapy, and no other commercially available formulation.

# Eight Cases from Our Files

*(By Dr. Gonzalez)*

In this section, I have included a total of eight case reports describing patients treated by us with the enzyme therapy. In each, the diagnosis has been confirmed by appropriate biopsy. All eight, at the time of initial presentation, had either poor prognosis or terminal disease by the standards of conventional oncology. For seven patients, all long-term survivors, I provide documentation confirming disease regression while each pursued only our therapy. In one case, a woman diagnosed with widely metastatic ovarian cancer, though we lack radiographic evidence of tumor shrinkage, her very long-term, 19-year survival seems proof enough of response. Overall, these case reports hopefully illustrate that the therapy continues to work effectively with poor prognosis malignant disease.

Since we are known for our success with pancreatic cancer, we decided to include three case histories of patients diagnosed with the adenocarcinoma form of the disease, still considered by most experts to be the malignancy with the worst overall prognosis. We have in addition written up one patient with metastatic islet cell carcinoma of the pancreas whose tumors regressed completely while under our care. True, patients with this subtype fare somewhat better than those with the exocrine variety, but we felt his complete response warranted inclusion in the series.

The remaining four consist of one patient diagnosed with breast cancer metastatic to the liver and brain; one with metastatic ovarian cancer; one with metastatic renal cell cancer; and finally, one with widely metastatic uterine carcinoma.

## PATIENT IK: *A 19–Year Survivor of Metastatic Breast Cancer*

Patient IK is a 64-year-old woman with a strong family history of breast cancer. She had previously been in good health when in the fall of 1986, routine mammography revealed a suspicious mass in the left breast, confirmed by biopsy as ductal carcinoma in situ. Although her surgeon suggested a modified radical mastectomy, at IK's insistence he performed a lumpectomy, removing only the cancerous tumor. Since she had no evidence of metastatic disease, her doctors did not recommend additional adjuvant treatment.

She did well until July 1989, when her physician detected a mass in the right breast on routine follow-up examination. She subsequently underwent excision of the right breast tumor along with a 3 cm right axillary mass, both of which proved to be infiltrated with poorly differentiated adenocarcinoma, estrogen and progesterone receptor negative. After surgery, an abdominal ultrasound revealed a density on the right lobe of the liver consistent with metastatic disease. A needle biopsy of the hepatic lesion confirmed metastatic cancer, and a bone scan showed "multiple focal areas of increased activity in the spine consistent with metastatic carcinoma."

IK then began chemotherapy with CAF, a very aggressive protocol which she tolerated poorly. In late 1989, after completing three cycles of the proposed six, she refused further treatment and for several months, did nothing before visiting Stanford in the spring of 1990 for a second opinion. There, after reviewing the previous biopsies and scans, the physicians concurred with the diagnosis of metastatic disease to the liver. The Stanford note reports "The diagnosis is confirmed and the liver involvement has been documented by the Stanford Pathology Laboratory."

Her doctor at Stanford recommended she immediately resume chemotherapy with CAF, but once again, IK refused to consider further conventional approaches. Instead, after learning of our work, she decided to pursue our program and was first seen in our office in April 1990.

She was quite ill at the time, very debilitated, with chronic pain in her liver. After returning home and beginning her regimen, the liver pain was so severe she required morphine for comfort. She also reported fatigue and malaise lasting many months, before she finally began to improve. When I saw her for a return evaluation in May 1991—a year after she had begun her nutritional protocol—she felt much stronger and her abdominal pains had largely resolved. Unfortunately, she began to feel so well that without my knowledge, she subsequently discontinued her protocol, assuming she was "cured." In early July 1991, she called me very distraught, having just suffered a grand mal seizure, and admitting she had been off her regimen for several months. A CT scan of the brain revealed a high-density epidural mass in the left sphenoidal ridge as well as a small low density area in the right temporoparietal region. The radiology report reads "Both areas were heterogeneously enhanced with contrast medium and appear to be metastatic brain lesions."

Her doctors immediately recommended radiation to the brain, which IK refused. Instead, she resumed her full nutritional program with renewed dedication, quickly improved and never experienced another seizure. Follow up CT scans of both the head and abdomen in April 1992, less than a year after her recurrence, were completely normal—the previously noted brain and liver tumors were gone. The report of the head CT reads "There is no mass or mass effect . . . There is no evidence of metastatic disease . . . Normal CT scan of the head." The summary of the abdominal scan states: "Normal CT scan of the abdomen."

Since that time, IK has had an up and down history on my program, with periods of good compliance and periods of less than good compliance, though her breast cancer never again recurred. I haven't seen her in my office in some years, but hear periodically that she is still doing well and still taking enzymes. I recently learned from another patient of mine who knows her well that as of June 2008 she appears to be in excellent health, now 19 years after her diagnosis of terminal metastatic breast cancer.

In her battle with cancer, IK served as her own "control"—when she followed the program she did well, when her compliance fell off, the cancer came back with a vengeance. The disease then completely regressed when adherence to therapy improved.

We usually tell new patients coming to us with a history of metastatic cancer that they need to follow their nutritional regimen indefinitely, never assuming they are completely free and clear. We think of cancer as a chronic degenerative disease, akin to diabetes, that can be managed successfully for years as long as patients follow their diet and take their enzymes. When compliance falls off, as in this case, cancer can return with resulting havoc. Renewed dedication to the treatment usually gets the situation back under control.

Regardless of her compliance lapses, IK's survival is extraordinary. As the medical literature documents, breast cancer, when metastatic to either the brain or liver, is a deadly disease. In a series of patients with brain metastases specifically, Lentzsch et al report a median survival of 23 weeks for those with more than one lesion, despite aggressive conventional treatment.[119] In a group of patients with at least one lesion receiving supportive care only, the authors describe a median survival of five weeks.

Eichbaum et al studied a group of 350 women with breast cancer that had metastasized to the liver.[120] The authors report a median survival, regardless of the conventional treatment given, of 14 months, somewhat better than the numbers for brain metastases, but still dismal.

In this case, with evidence of liver, brain and bone metastases—as deadly a combination as can be imagined—IK's 19-year survival is remarkable.

## PATIENT AL: *A 19-Year Survivor Of Metastatic Ovarian Cancer*

Patient AL, prior to developing cancer, had a long history of neuromuscular symptoms dating to 1979, when she first developed a mass in her left calf associated with muscle pain, atrophy, and numbness. In the intervening years, as the symptoms worsened she consulted numerous physicians at numerous centers. Though multiple muscle biopsies revealed no underlying cause for her distress, she was nonetheless treated empirically and unsuccessfully with a variety of drugs including prednisone. In 1985, she sought another evaluation at the Mayo Clinic, where a muscle biopsy confirmed polymyositis. After she was also diagnosed with motor and sensory neuropathy type II, AL began another course of prednisone with little improvement, followed by six months on Imuran. The latter drug did nothing for her disease, but did lead to weight gain, insomnia and anxiety.

As her symptoms worsened, AL, who knew of my work from a family member, decided to seek treatment with me for her neuromuscular problems. When she first came to my office in 1989, she had been off all medications for some three years, during which time her symptoms of weakness, nerve pain, and numbness continued to progress. When I first saw her, she had no gynecological problems other than the history of a hysterectomy for uterine fibroids.

I designed a protocol to treat this patient's muscle and neurological problems, without the high doses of enzymes we prescribe for those diagnosed with cancer. Subsequently, AL complied well with her program, and when I saw her for a return visit in August 1989, she reported her condition that had previously deteriorated without respite over a ten year period had improved significantly. She described a "20%" overall gain in motor strength and calf thickness, a marker her previous doctors had used to track her decline. The proximal muscle weakness in both legs had reversed to the point she could stand from a sitting position for the first time in years. However, after detecting a small pelvic mass on exam, I told her she needed to follow up with a gynecological evaluation upon returning home.

Some weeks later, in early fall, an ultrasound revealed a 7 x 8 cm cystic lesion posterior to the bladder. In early November 1989, at the Moffitt

Cancer Center in Tampa, during exploratory laparotomy she was found to have extensive malignant disease throughout her pelvis and abdomen. Her surgeon proceeded with bilateral oophorectomy, omentectomy, and extensive resection of pelvic, periaortic, and precaval lymph nodes. The pathology report describes "Omentum diffusely infiltrated by papillary serous carcinoma" of ovarian origin, as well as tumor in both ovaries and both fallopian tubes. All 21 of 21 nodes evaluated were positive for cancer, and peritoneal washings revealed "metastatic adenocarcinoma consistent with ovarian primary."

After surgery, AL met with an oncologist who strongly recommended intensive chemotherapy, but she decided to refuse all conventional treatment, instead choosing to begin the cancer version of my therapy. At that point, I redesigned her regimen to include high doses of pancreatic enzymes throughout the day.

In December 1989 her oncologist wrote a summary note to me, which accompanied the records of her recent hospitalization. In his letter, he states:

> She is diagnosed as having a Stage IIIC Grade I papillary serous cystadenocarcinoma of the ovary. I have recommended that she receive chemotherapy. She would be a candidate for GOG Protocol 104 intravenous Cisplatinum and Cyclophosphamide versus intraperitoneal Cisplatinum and Cyclophosphamide. Mrs.—— unfortunately did not wish to pursue the idea of chemotherapy . . .

She thereafter followed her program diligently for six years. By the mid-1990s, her muscle weakness began to progress once again, making return trips to New York difficult, though she continued on the regimen and we worked together by phone. We last spoke in early 2009, when she reported her biggest problem was her ongoing neuromuscular weakness in her legs, requiring she use a walker for ambulation. She suddenly passed away in the spring of 2009 from pneumonia, at age 87. At the time, she was cancer-free, nearly 20 years from her diagnosis of extensive ovarian malignancy.

In the text *Cancer: Principles & Practice of Oncology,* the authors report that patients such as this diagnosed with extensive stage III disease have a five-year survival rate in the range of 15–20%.[29(p1604)] In this case, the disease did extend into the upper abdomen at the time of diagnosis, a warning sign of a poor prognosis. Furthermore, these survival statistics refer to patients treated with aggressive chemotherapy, which AL refused, choosing to follow only my regimen. Her prolonged disease-free survival can only be attributed to her nutritional program.

## PATIENT DQ: *a 16-Year Survivor Of Renal Cell Carcinoma*

Patient DQ had a past medical history pertinent for celiac disease, gout, and chronic borderline anemia. He had otherwise been in good health when in October 1990 his primary physician noted an abdominal mass during a routine yearly physical examination. Subsequent MRI and CT scan studies revealed a 14 cm tumor in the left kidney, with no evidence of metastases. After a chest X-ray and bone scan were both clear, in late October 1990 DQ underwent exploratory laparotomy and left nephrectomy. The tumor was diagnosed as renal cell carcinoma, with one adjacent node positive for invasive cancer.

DQ was then referred to a major New York medical center for additional evaluation and treatment. In December 1990 he agreed to enter a clinical trial testing alpha-interferon, an immune stimulant, for patients diagnosed with kidney cancer. After repeat chest and abdominal CT scans showed no evidence of residual or recurrent disease, DQ then began an eight-cycle course of intensive interferon, which he completed in August of 1991.

Only three months later, in November 1991, DQ noticed a lump in the left parietal-occipital region of the skull that rapidly enlarged over a period of several days, quickly reaching the size of a small lemon. In early December 1991 needle aspiration of the mass confirmed "Adenocarcinoma, consistent with metastatic renal tubular carcinoma."

A subsequent CT scan of the head indicated that the tumor had penetrated through the skull into the cranium, as the report states:

> There is a lytic lesion within the left parietal bone with an associated enhancing soft tissue mass, consistent with a metastasis. There is intracranial extension of the enhancing soft tissue, as well as extension into the subcutaneous tissues of the left parietal scalp.

A bone scan showed "a large focal area of increased radiopharmaceutical uptake with a photopenic center consistent with metastatic disease in the left occipital region of the skull." A CT scan of the chest revealed

"Small nodule at the left lung base . . . which may be an area of fibrosis as described. Two other smaller densities in the middle lobe and the left lower lobe as described of questionable significance." However, these lung findings had not been reported on the chest CT of December 1990.

DQ then began a one-month course of radiation to the skull mass, totaling 4000 rads, but despite the treatment the tumor regressed only marginally. DQ, now told he had incurable disease, began looking into alternative approaches, learned of my work and decided to pursue my protocol. When we first met in January 1992, only a week after he had finished radiation, DQ reported significantly diminished energy, along with a 20-pound weight loss occurring during the previous six weeks. On exam, I immediately noticed a lemon-sized mass sticking out of his skull in the left parietal area.

Shortly thereafter, DQ began his nutritional protocol, complied well, and within weeks reported a significant improvement in his energy and general well being, accompanied by a 20-pound weight gain. After three months on therapy, the previously noted large skull mass completely resolved. A repeat bone scan in June 1993, after DQ had completed some 16 months of treatment, revealed "No evidence of bony metastatic disease." Not only had the lesion disappeared, but the underlying skull had healed. Unfortunately DQ eventually passed away in July 2007 at 83 years old after suffering a stroke, I believe caused by damage from the radiation given in early 1992. He nonetheless survived 15 years, for most of the time in excellent health while following his nutritional program.

Several points need mentioning. For stage IV metastatic renal cell carcinoma, a very deadly disease, *Cancer: Principles & Practice of Oncology* reports a median survival of only 50 days despite treatment.[29(p1369)] This neoplasm resists not only chemotherapy and immunotherapy, but radiation as well. In this case, DQ's doctors suggested radiation not as a potential cure but as palliation, hoping to slow the spread of the tumor into the brain. In any event, the response was negligible. While oncologists report that at times the benefit of radiation therapy might continue for up to two months, DQ showed significant response only after the third month on his nutritional program. Furthermore, although his radiologists initially downplayed the findings on the chest CT in late 1991, in retrospect these lesions may have indicated the beginnings of explosive spread.

**PATIENT LR:** *A 15-year Survivor Of Metastatic Pancreatic Cancer*

Patient LR, like so many of my patients, has an unusual background, with a graduate degree, study abroad, and expertise in art. Before we first met, he had worked successfully in business for many years. His very devoted wife had earned a Ph.D. in literature and had, before retirement, worked as a college professor.

He had been in good health when in July 1991, at age 70, a routine chest x-ray at the time of his yearly physical revealed a small right lung nodule suspicious for possible malignancy. A repeat x-ray in August 1991 again demonstrated "a parenchymal nodule in the right mid lung . . . " CT scan studies of the chest in late August 1991 confirmed a "6 millimeter nodule in peripheral lateral aspect of right upper lobe. It is consistent with bronchogenic carcinoma, metastatic lesion or granuloma . . . " In addition, the radiologist noted "an enlarged lymph node posterior to the ascending thoracic aorta . . . "

A CT scan of the brain in early September 1991 was clear, but a CT scan of the abdomen revealed extensive disease throughout:

> There are about 4 lesions in the upper right lobe of the liver . . . An ultrasound examination is recommended for further evaluation . . .

> There is a round enlargement of the right adrenal gland up to 2 cm in diameter. There is also what appears to be diffuse enlargement of the left adrenal . . . Both these findings are suspicious for metastatic disease. There is a mass in what may be the cephalad portion of the head of the pancreas or it is a mass or adenopathy just adjacent to the head. The mass measures about 4.5 cm in its greater diameter . . .

A bone scan the same day demonstrated: "Abnormal activity of the right hip and right shoulder suggesting metastatic disease . . . "

Though the situation appeared dismal, the patient's doctors still suggested biopsy studies to confirm the diagnosis of cancer and help determine the most likely primary site. After reviewing the scans, they decided the lung lesion to be most accessible for tissue sampling, so in late September 1991 LR was admitted to his local hospital for mediastinoscopy and a limited right thoracotomy. In his admission note, the surgeon reports that the patient's presentation seemed most consistent with pancreatic cancer that had metastasized to the lung, not lung cancer that had spread into the abdomen:

> At some point, I suspect he will require oncology and radiation medicine consultation for what is most likely a pancreatic carcinoma with multiple metastatic lesions.

The lung nodule proved to be adenocarcinoma, as the pathology report describes:

> Right upper lobe lung nodule, biopsy: Infiltrative moderately differentiated adenocarcinoma.

After surgery, an ultrasound again revealed the liver lesions:

> Areas consistent with metastatic involvement of the liver, the largest of which is approximately 3.4 to 4 cm in maximal dimension near the hilus. The second is just under 2 cm in the right lobe and possibly a third smaller one in the right lobe.

With the evaluation complete, LR was told he had metastatic pancreatic cancer, perhaps two months to live, and that neither chemotherapy nor radiation would be of benefit. But instead of going home to die, he and his wife decided to take the situation into their own hands. They both read voraciously about cancer, nutrition, and alternatives. He began ingesting large numbers of supplements, including vitamin C, vitamin E, even pancreatic enzymes after reading an article discussing our work. He switched his eating habits to a largely plant-based, raw diet, and began juicing intensively, with his wife's help. When he felt sufficiently recovered from surgery, he decided to consult with me.

When I first saw LR in December 1991, despite his prognosis he seemed determined to fight his disease. Subsequently he complied well and within a year his general health had improved substantially. A CT scan of the abdomen in February 1993—some 15 months after his initial diagnosis—showed no change in any of the lesions. Though technically the cancer hadn't improved, the disease hadn't advanced and he was still alive.

After that set of scans LR told me he wanted no more testing. Since he had already long outlived his doctors' dismal predictions by that point, he explained to me that he did not care what the scans might show nor would he change his treatment whatever the findings. So he continued his therapy, enjoying with his wife the retirement for which they had long planned.

In 1997, after he had followed his nutritional protocol for five years, he agreed—with some pleading from me—to allow radiographic studies. A CT of the abdomen in March 1997 showed two mildly enlarged adrenal glands and a single, very small, less than 1 cm mass in the dome of the liver. The other large liver lesions were gone. The radiologist in his report described the pancreas as normal—the previously documented large tumor had simply disappeared:

> The liver demonstrated a single small hypodense area in the dome of the liver which has the appearance of a cyst, measuring well less than 1 cm. A metastatic lesion is still a possibility especially in view of the patient's history of lung cancer and adrenal mass . . . The adrenal glands are both abnormal . . . The pancreas, the spleen and the kidneys are within normal limits. There is no evidence of periaortic lymphadenopathy.

Then 16 months later, in July of 1998, nearly seven years after his diagnosis, LR agreed to undergo repeat scanning. The radiologist describes the findings as follows:

> Reading the report from the 1993 study it sounded like the patient had obvious metastatic disease and the largest structure being a large porta hepatis and peripancreatic mass. No such masses are seen today. There is no adenopathy. The adrenals are prominent and there are two very small liver lesions that cannot be characterized because of their small size.

Thereafter, LR complied with his program and continued doing well until he was involved in a serious automobile accident in 2004. Unfortunately, he required lengthy rehabilitation, followed by life in an assisted care facility. His wife, three years older, no longer able to care for herself at 87 years old, also entered an assisted care facility, where she died. At last contact LR was still alive, more than 15 years since his diagnosis of terminal metastatic pancreatic adenocarcinoma.

His case does not require much discussion. He was diagnosed appropriately with terminal cancer and given two months to live. He did his program, the tumors went away, and he survived.

**PATIENT CI:** *A 14-Year Survivor Of Metastatic Pancreatic Cancer*

Patient CI had been previously very healthy when he first developed chronic heartburn, gradual weight loss, and persistent diarrhea throughout the summer of 1992. In August of that year, he became suddenly very weak and short of breath; when his local doctor found him to be severely anemic, he was hospitalized for a transfusion and diagnostic evaluation. Endoscopy showed multiple stomach ulcers, assumed to be the source of the blood loss. Additional testing revealed elevated blood levels of gastrin, a hormone which stimulates the parietal cells of the stomach to secrete hydrochloric acid. High serum gastrin, often associated with multiple ulcerations such as in this patient's case, usually warns of a hormone-secreting pancreatic tumor. However, despite extensive searching, no such lesion could be found, so after prescribing Prilosec, his doctors sent CI home.

On the medication he actually did fairly well, with no further bouts of severe anemia until October 1994 when his gastrin levels on routine blood testing were again elevated. This time around, a CT scan did show a 6 to 7 cm mass in the retroperitoneal area of the abdomen. After a series of delays, he underwent exploratory abdominal surgery in March 1995 at a local hospital, at which time his surgeon discovered a very large pancreatic tumor. Because of its size and degree of infiltration throughout the organ, the mass could not be removed, though it was biopsied. In addition, a metastatic lesion at the base of the liver was resected, as described in the operative note:

> There was however a large uncinate process grossly clinically involved with tumor. Also, the whole head of the pancreas clinically was involved with tumor as well. Lateral to the head of the pancreas on the other side of the SMV [superior mesenteric vein] and the neck and body region was also palpable tumor.
>
> Palpation and exploration of the porta hepatis revealed approximately a 3 cm mass noted . . . This was sharply dissected and free [sic] and sent to pathology for quick frozen section . . .

The pathology report confirmed, in both the pancreatic and portal lymph node biopsies, "carcinoid-islet cell tumor."

After recovering from surgery, CI decided to travel for a second opinion to the Mayo Clinic, where he was seen in May 1995. At Mayo, the original slides were reviewed, with the diagnosis of islet cell carcinoma verified. At the time, the consulting oncologist recommended no additional therapy as the official Mayo note reads:

> I briefly discussed the case with my surgical colleague, Dr. ——. He did not feel that any further surgical intervention was warranted at this time. A Whipple procedure would be entirely palliative at this time. The patient may eventually come to a bypass procedure as there is some bile duct dilatation on CT scan. We discussed the fact that there is no good evidence for benefit from radiotherapy . . . I discussed with him the role of chemotherapy in patients with islet cell carcinoma . . . there is no evidence that earlier treatment will show improved response and survival. Given his asymptomatic state, I did not recommend any intervention at this time . . .

Initially, CI continued only on his Prilosec, but by early 1996, not content to wait until the disease progressed, he began investigating alternative cancer therapies. After learning of my work, he first came to my office in March 1996 and subsequently proved to be determined, very diligent and very disciplined with his nutritional regimen.

In June 1997, a little over a year after he first began treatment, a follow-up CT scan revealed "no significant change in the appearance of the patient's pancreatic mass since previous examinations." The tumor was still there, but no bigger.

For several years, since he felt so well, he avoided any testing until agreeing to another scan in September 2002. The official report stated:

> Findings: Images of the pancreas demonstrate no mass lesions. The liver, spleen adrenal glands and kidneys are unremarkable.

*Impression:*
    1. Normal CT scan of the abdomen.

The large tumor in his pancreas had simply gone away. A more recent scan again confirmed resolution of his once extensive disease, and today, 13 years after beginning his nutritional therapy, CI continues on his program and continues doing well.

This is not a complicated case. At surgery CI was found to have unresectable disease that had metastasized to the porta hepatis lymph nodes. Biopsies of the large unresectable pancreatic mass and the metastatic lesion revealed islet cell carcinoma, findings confirmed at the Mayo Clinic. CI then began my program, followed it faithfully, his tumors went away, and he remains cancer free and in excellent health, nearly 14 years from his original diagnosis.

### PATIENT RB: *An 8-Year Survivor Of Metastatic Pancreatic Cancer*

In November 2000, Patient RB first reported a gradual 25-pound weight loss to her local physician. A CT scan of the abdomen in early December 2000 revealed a 3.4 cm mass in the head of the pancreas, but no evidence of metastatic disease. A subsequent CT scan-guided needle biopsy in February 2001 confirmed a "Poorly differentiated adenocarcinoma, ductal type," the most aggressive form of pancreatic cancer. The slides were also sent to the Mayo Clinic, where the consulting pathologist confirmed the diagnosis of adenocarcinoma.

Since the cancer appeared to be localized, the patient's physicians suggested aggressive surgery, but she decided the risks were too great, the potential benefits too meager, to warrant such an approach. She subsequently learned of our treatment regimen and in March 2001 consulted with Dr. Isaacs. In April 2001, a month after she began her nutrition treatment, repeat CT scans revealed a 3.2 cm mass in the head of the pancreas, with no evidence of metastatic disease.

A follow-up CT scan performed in January 2002, some ten months after she began treatment with Dr. Isaacs, indicated a 3.0 x 3.0 cm mass in the head of the pancreas, smaller compared to the scan of April 2001. The next CT in July 2003, after RB had followed her nutritional regimen for more than two years, showed a 3.16 x 2.6 cm mass in the head of the pancreas, and a scan not quite a year later revealed a 3 x 2.8 cm lesion.

RB, now an eight year survivor, currently reports excellent health despite her original poor prognosis. In her case, the CT scans show perhaps some slight shrinkage in her tumor, but no spread. Given the aggressive nature of pancreatic adenocarcinoma in general, and the virulent nature of the poorly differentiated variety diagnosed in this case, its tendency to metastasize and kill within a year even when aggressively treated, this patient's course has truly been remarkable. She has been able to avoid extensive surgery, chemotherapy, and radiation while enjoying excellent health.

As a side note, we do find in our practice that though tumors often disappear—as in the previously discussed cases of pancreatic cancer—at times they seem to stabilize, sometimes for many years.

## PATIENT CX: *An 8-Year Survivor Of Metastatic Pancreatic Cancer*

In January 2001, Patient CX, with a long history of GERD (gastroe-sophageal reflux disease) decided to undergo elective laparoscopic surgery for correction of what was presumed to be a simple hiatal hernia. During the procedure, his physician discovered "multiple umbilicated, white, firm, and gritty tumors in both the right and left lobes of the liver, apparently occupying approximately 50% of the volume of the liver."

A biopsy of one of the liver lesions confirmed "poorly differentiated metastatic carcinoma," with some "neuroendocrine differentiation." The final pathological diagnosis reads:

> Liver needle biopsy
>
> Positive for malignancy, favor metastatic adenocarcinoma.

After surgery, a CT scan of the chest, abdomen, and pelvis revealed a large 6.5 × 3.7 cm mass in the tail of the pancreas, with "diffuse hepatic metastases." The radiologist wrote "This likely represents primary pancreatic adenocarcinoma."

The patient subsequently met with an oncologist at Barnes Hospital in St. Louis who suggested aggressive chemotherapy with cisplatin and etoposide for four cycles, though he admitted that even with chemotherapy, the disease would ultimately progress and prove deadly. Before agreeing to the treatment, in February 2001 CX traveled to Memorial Sloan-Kettering in New York for a second opinion. There, after reviewing the slides, the Memorial pathologists confirmed a very aggressive pancreatic carcinoma. The consulting oncologist then proposed the same chemotherapy protocol that had been previously recommended but again warned that even with aggressive treatment, CX might live at most two years. Chemotherapy, as he had been told before, might shrink his tumors and prolong his life, but would not provide a long-term solution.

At the time of the Memorial consultation, CX was not doing well clinically, as reported in the notes from the visit:

The patient has significant fatigue, takes naps usually by the end of the afternoon. He does notice recent onset back pain which is alleviated with pain pills. He has significant nausea without vomiting . . . .He does have occasional palpitations but denies flushing. He notes mildly decreased appetite and has had an approximately ten-pound weight loss.

After returning home, CX began the proposed course of chemotherapy in February 2001 under the direction of his local oncologist. After the first cycle, a CT scan in February 2001 indicated some response to chemotherapy:

As on the prior examination, there is a low attenuation mass within the tail of the pancreas. The mass is smaller in size, measuring 6.4 cm x 3.0 cm on the current examination . . . .on today's study there are innumerable low attenuation lesions throughout the liver, measuring up to 2 cm in diameter, consistent with metastatic disease . . .

After the second cycle of chemotherapy, a repeat CT scan in March 2001 showed: "Marked improvement in numerous liver metastases with a decreased [sic] in size as well of the pancreatic tail mass."

CX completed the first three cycles of chemotherapy without much difficulty, but during the fourth round he became so ill the drugs had to be discontinued in April 2001. Then, after learning about our work, he decided to forgo further chemotherapy, choosing to proceed with our treatment.

I first saw CX in my office in May 2001, four weeks after his last round of drugs. Thereafter CX proved to be very compliant with his nutritional regimen and within months he reported significant improvement in his general health. His many symptoms, including persistent debilitating fatigue, had resolved.

In February 2002, after Patient CX had completed 10 months on the therapy, a CT scan of the abdomen demonstrated multiple small lesions in the liver which had been seen on previous scans, as discussed in the official note:

202 The Trophoblast and the Origins of Cancer

1. Multiple tiny lesions in the liver, all less than 3 mm in size. Some of these lesions have been noted on prior studies which were obtained at slightly larger collimation [*calibration*] and have not changed since the previous studies.
2. No pancreatic lesion.
3. No abdomen or pelvic lesion.

At that point, I made several adjustments in his regimen. A subsequent CT scan in October 2002, some 17 months after he had first begun his nutritional therapy, confirmed that all the liver tumors were gone. The report states:

1. No pancreatic lesion identified.
2. Multiple tiny lesions in the liver seen on the prior examination are not identified on today's study.

Follow up scans in March 2003 and June 2004 also documented complete resolution of his disease, and his most recent scan in early 2009 again showed no evidence of recurrent malignancy. At this time, he has been following his program for nearly eight years, remains cancer-free and in excellent health despite the original diagnosis of very advanced and very terminal pancreatic carcinoma.

This case is very straightforward. Though aggressive chemotherapy did shrink the primary pancreatic lesion as well as the liver tumors, the disease did not completely regress on drug treatment. Furthermore, the experts Patient CX consulted at Barnes and Memorial Sloan-Kettering both warned him even if he showed some response, the benefit would be short-lived. Not even the most fanatical oncologist claims chemotherapy cures pancreatic carcinoma metastatic to the liver. Finally, it was only on his nutritional regimen that the tumors regressed completely and stayed that way.

### PATIENT JK: *A 15-Year Survivor Of Metastatic Uterine Cancer*

Patient JK is a 62-year-old woman who had been in good health when in the fall of 1990 she required hospitalization for two episodes of deep venous thrombosis. She was placed on Coumadin, but shortly thereafter suffered an episode of severe vaginal hemorrhage. When the bleeding persisted, in December 1990 she underwent a D&C, which revealed endometrial carcinoma. After a CT scan in January 1991 showed extensive abdominal and pelvic lymphadenopathy, she underwent a total abdominal hysterectomy with bilateral salpingo-oophorectomy.

The pathology report describes endometrial adenocarcinoma with areas of squamous differentiation, high nuclear grade (FIGO grade III), and papillary serous carcinoma, one of the most lethal of uterine malignancies. The tumor had spread to the left ovary, obliterating the fimbriated end of the left Fallopian tube. Biopsies of the peritoneal cul-de-sac as well as the rectal serosa confirmed metastatic disease, and due to the extent of spread, her doctors warned of a very poor prognosis.

Postoperatively, JK met with a radiation oncologist who insisted treatment begin at once but first, JK decided to consult with a second oncologist in a Southern tertiary care center. Again, radiation was aggressively pushed as essential to delay spread of her aggressive disease. However, JK decided to refuse all conventional treatments, instead choosing to medicate herself with a variety of nutritional supplements including high dose vitamin C and red clover tea.

An abdominal MRI in March 1991 showed a "decrease in degree of periaortic lymphadenopathy with persistent evidence of matted lymph nodes . . . " Pelvic MRI documented "decrease in the degree of diffuse pelvic lympadenopathy although there is persistent evidence of pelvic mass lesion most notable in the left hemipelvis. There is evidence of surgical defect presumably from previous hysterectomy . . . " So with surgery and her self-prescribed nutritional regimen, there had been improvement, though clearly extensive disease remained.

About that time, after learning of our work, JK decided to pursue my therapy. When first evaluated in my office in April 1991, she reported persistent fatigue, a substantial recent weight loss of 15 pounds, "terrible night sweats," and poor sleep.

JK subsequently followed her regimen with great determination. Seven months later, in December 1991, repeat MRIs showed no change in the periaortic lymphadenopathy as compared with the study of March 1991, but significant regression of the pelvic adenopathy and the mass in the left hemipelvis. The official report states:

> Compared to the study of 3–91, there is continued improvement with near complete resolution of previously seen pelvic lymphadenopathy. Currently, there is no appreciable residual mass lesion present within the left hemipelvis . . . .

Thereafter, JK continued her nutritional program diligently, with reported improvement in her general health. MRI studies of the abdomen and pelvis in January 1993, after she had completed some 20 months on therapy, indicated that the previously noted extensive disease had completely resolved. The written report of the pelvic scan states: "There is no identified pelvic lymphadenopathy." The abdominal MRI revealed: "There is no evidence of significant periaortic or periportal lymphadenopathy."

MRI studies completed 14 months later, in March 1994 confirmed: "There is no distinct evidence of metastatic or recurrent disease."

JK followed her regimen faithfully until early 1997, when I last spoke with her. At that time, six years from her diagnosis of metastatic aggressive endometrial cancer, she remained disease-free and generally in good health. She subsequently continued her therapy in a reduced way, and now, more than 17 years from diagnosis, I have heard she is alive and apparently doing well.

This case is, like the others, straightforward: the patient was diagnosed with metastatic papillary serous carcinoma, one of the most deadly subtypes of uterine cancer. The surgeon could not excise all the visible cancer, as MRI studies after surgery documented. She then experienced complete regression of her advanced disease while following her nutritional program only, and was alive and well at last report 15 years later.

# References

(1) Murray MJ, Lessey BA. Embryo implantation and tumor metastasis: common pathways of invasion and angiogenesis. *Semin Reprod Endocrinol.* 1999;17:275–290.

(2) Ferretti C, Bruni L, Dangles-Marie V, Pecking AP, Bellet D. Molecular circuits shared by placental and cancer cells, and their implications in the proliferative, invasive and migratory capacities of trophoblasts. *Hum Reprod Update.* 2007;13:121–141.

(3) Beard J. *The Enzyme Treatment of Cancer.* London: Chatto and Windus; 1911.

(4) Carlson BM. *Human Embryology & Developmental Biology.* 2nd ed. St. Louis, MO: Mosby; 1999.

(5) Norwitz ER, Schust DJ, Fisher SJ. Implantation and the survival of early pregnancy. *N Engl J Med.* 2001;345:1400–1408.

(6) Cohen M, Bischof P. Factors regulating trophoblast invasion. *Gynecol Obstet Invest.* 2007;64:126–130.

(7) Lunghi L, Ferretti ME, Medici S, Biondi C, Vesce F. Control of human trophoblast function. *Reprod Biol Endocrinol.* 2007;5:6.

(8) Cross JC. Formation of the placenta and extraembryonic membranes. *Ann N Y Acad Sci.* 1998;857:23–32.:23–32.

(9) Cross JC, Werb Z, Fisher SJ. Implantation and the placenta: key pieces of the development puzzle. *Science.* 1994;266:1508–1518.

(10) Bischof P, Meisser A, Campana A. Biochemistry and molecular biology of trophoblast invasion. *Ann N Y Acad Sci.* 2001;943:157–162.

(11) Bhagavan NV. *Medical Biochemistry.* Boston, MA: Jones and Bartlett Publishers International; 1992.

(12) Arias JI, Aller MA, Arias J. Cancer cell: using inflammation to invade the host. *Mol Cancer.* 2007;6:29.

(13) Kasper DL, Braunwald E, Fauci AS, Hauser SL, Longo DL, Jameson JL, editors. *Harrison's Principles of Internal Medicine.* 16th ed. New York, NY: McGraw-Hill; 2005.

(14) Anin SA, Vince G, Quenby S. Trophoblast invasion. *Hum Fertil (Camb ).* 2004;7:169–174.

(15) Kliman H. From trophoblast to human placenta. http://www.med.yale.edu/obgyn/kliman/placenta/articles/EOR_Placenta/Trophtoplacenta.html. Accessed June 18, 2008.

(16) Robbins SL, Cotran RS. *Pathologic Basis of Disease*. 2nd ed. Philadelphia, PA: W.B. Saunders; 1979.

(17) Wells M. The pathology of gestational trophoblastic disease: recent advances. *Pathology*. 2007;39:88–96.

(18) Cross JC, Flannery ML, Blanar MA et al. Hxt encodes a basic helix-loop-helix transcription factor that regulates trophoblast cell development. *Development*. 1995;121:2513–2523.

(19) Janatpour MJ, Utset MF, Cross JC et al. A repertoire of differentially expressed transcription factors that offers insight into mechanisms of human cytotrophoblast differentiation. *Dev Genet*. 1999;25:146–157.

(20) Scott IC, Anson-Cartwright L, Riley P, Reda D, Cross JC. The HAND1 basic helix-loop-helix transcription factor regulates trophoblast differentiation via multiple mechanisms. *Mol Cell Biol*. 2000; 20:530–541.

(21) Hay DC, Sutherland L, Clark J, Burdon T. Oct-4 knockdown induces similar patterns of endoderm and trophoblast differentiation markers in human and mouse embryonic stem cells. *Stem Cells*. 2004;22:225–235.

(22) Ezashi T, Ghosh D, Roberts RM. Repression of Ets-2-induced transactivation of the tau interferon promoter by Oct-4. *Mol Cell Biol*. 2001;21:7883–7891.

(23) Cross JC, Anson-Cartwright L, Scott IC. Transcription factors underlying the development and endocrine functions of the placenta. *Recent Prog Horm Res*. 2002;57:221–34.

(24) Cross JC. Genetic insights into trophoblast differentiation and placental morphogenesis. *Semin Cell Dev Biol*. 2000;11:105–113.

(25) Janatpour MJ, McMaster MT, Genbacev O et al. Id-2 regulates critical aspects of human cytotrophoblast differentiation, invasion and migration. *Development*. 2000;127: 549–558.

(26) Cellular differentiation. http://en.wikipedia.org/wiki/Cellular_differentiation. Accessed May 12, 2008.

(27) Braunwald E, Hauser SL, Fauci AS, Longo DL, Kasper DL, Jameson JL, editors. *Harrison's Principles of Internal Medicine*. 15th ed. New York, NY: McGraw-Hill; 2001.

(28) Staff AC. An introduction to cell migration and invasion. *Scand J Clin Lab Invest*. 2001;61:257–268.

(29) DeVita VT, Jr., Hellman S, Rosenberg SA, editors. *Cancer: Principles & Practice of Oncology*. 6th ed. Philadelphia, PA: Lippincott Williams & Wilkins; 2001.

(30) Cross JC, Hemberger M, Lu Y et al. Trophoblast functions, angiogenesis and remodeling of the maternal vasculature in the placenta. *Mol Cell Endocrinol*. 2002;187:207–212.

(31) Miller SJ, Lavker RM, Sun TT. Interpreting epithelial cancer biology in the context of stem cells: tumor properties and therapeutic implications. *Biochim Biophys Acta*. 2005;1756:25–52.

(32) O'Day DH. Saga of the sex cells. http://www.utm.utoronto.ca/~w3bio380/pdf/lecture2.pdf. Accessed June 18, 2008.

(33) Shimkin MB. *Science and Cancer*. Washington, DC: U.S. Department of Health, Education and Welfare, Public Health Service, National Cancer Institute; 1964.

(34) Parthenogenesis. http://www.infoplease.com/ce6/sci/A0837738.html. Accessed June 18, 2008.

(35) DeVita VT, Jr., Hellman S, Rosenberg SA, editors. *Cancer: Principles & Practice of Oncology*. 5th ed. Philadelphia, PA: Lippincott-Raven Publishers; 1997.

(36) Balkwill F, Mantovani A. Inflammation and cancer: back to Virchow? *Lancet*. 2001;357: 539–545.

(37) Turnpenny L, Brickwood S, Spalluto CM et al. Derivation of human embryonic germ cells: an alternative source of pluripotent stem cells. *Stem Cells*. 2003;21:598–609.

(38) The stem cell. http://stemcells.nih.gov/info/scireport/chapter1.asp. Accessed June 18, 2008.

(39) Stem cell. http://en.wikipedia.org/wiki/Stem_cell. Accessed May 6, 2008.

(40) Guenechea G, Gan OI, Dorrell C, Dick JE. Distinct classes of human stem cells that differ in proliferative and self-renewal potential. *Nat Immunol*. 2001;2:75–82.

(41) The adult stem cell. http://stemcells.nih.gov/info/scireport/chapter4.asp. Accessed June 18, 2008.

(42) Stem cells and diseases. http://stemcells.nih.gov/info/health.asp. Accessed June 18, 2008.

(43) Leger CS, Nevill TJ. Hematopoietic stem cell transplantation: a primer for the primary care physician. *CMAJ*. 2004;170:1569–1577.

(44) Zikos P, Van Lint MT, Frassoni F et al. Low transplant mortality in allogeneic bone marrow transplantation for acute myeloid leukemia: a randomized study of low-dose cyclosporin versus low-dose cyclosporin and low-dose methotrexate. *Blood*. 1998;91:3503–3508.

(45) Hematopoietic stem cell transplantation. http://en.wikipedia.org/wiki/Stem_cell_transplant. Accessed June 18, 2008.

(46) Alison MR, Poulsom R, Jeffery R et al. Hepatocytes from non-hepatic adult stem cells. *Nature*. 2000;406:257.

(47) Theise ND, Nimmakayalu M, Gardner R et al. Liver from bone marrow in humans. *Hepatology*. 2000;32:11–16.

(48) Turnpenny L, Spalluto CM, Perrett RM et al. Evaluating human embryonic germ cells: concord and conflict as pluripotent stem cells. *Stem Cells*. 2006;24:212–220.

(49) Beard J. The system of branchial sense organs and their associated ganglia in Ichthyopsida. *Quart J Microsc Soc*. 1885;11:52–90.

(50) Bonnet D, Dick JE. Human acute myeloid leukemia is organized as a hierarchy that originates from a primitive hematopoietic cell. *Nat Med*. 1997;3:730–737.

(51) Dick JE. Acute myeloid leukemia stem cells. *Ann N Y Acad Sci*. 2005;1044:1–5.

(52) Dick JE, Lapidot T. Biology of normal and acute myeloid leukemia stem cells. *Int J Hematol*. 2005;82:389–396.

(53) Dontu G, Al-Hajj M, Abdallah WM, Clarke MF, Wicha MS. Stem cells in normal breast development and breast cancer. *Cell Prolif*. 2003;36 Suppl 1:59–72.

(54) Pobojewski S. U-M scientists find "stem cells" in human breast cancer. http://www.cancer.med.umich.edu/news/stemcell.htm. Accessed June 18, 2008.

(55)  Nelson R. Brain-cancer stem cells may drive tumour formation. *Lancet Neurol.* 2005;4:17.

(56)  Singh SK, Hawkins C, Clarke ID et al. Identification of human brain tumour initiating cells. *Nature.* 2004;432:396–401.

(57)  Clarke MF, Dick JE, Dirks PB et al. Cancer stem cells—perspectives on current status and future directions: AACR Workshop on cancer stem cells. *Cancer Res.* 2006;66:9339–9344.

(58)  Wicha MS, Liu S, Dontu G. Cancer stem cells: an old idea—a paradigm shift. *Cancer Res.* 2006;66:1883–1890.

(59)  Li C, Heidt DG, Dalerba P et al. Identification of pancreatic cancer stem cells. *Cancer Res.* 2007;67:1030–1037.

(60)  Friel AM, Sergent PA, Patnaude C et al. Functional analyses of the cancer stem cell-like properties of human endometrial tumor initiating cells. *Cell Cycle.* 2008;7:242–249.

(61)  Growing evidence supports stem cell hypothesis of cancer. *Oncol News Int.* 2006;15: 24–25.

(62)  Acevedo HF, Hartsock RJ, Maroon JC. Detection of membrane-associated human chorionic gonadotropin and its subunits on human cultured cancer cells of the nervous system. *Cancer Detect Prev.* 1997;21:295–303.

(63)  Krichevsky A, Birken S, O'Connor J et al. Development, characterization, and application of monoclonal antibodies to the native and synthetic beta COOH-terminal portion of human chorionic gonadotropin (hCG) that distinguish between the native and desialylated forms of hCG. *Endocrinology.* 1994;134:1139–1145.

(64)  Acevedo HF, Krichevsky A, Campbell-Acevedo EA, Galyon JC, Buffo MJ, Hartsock RJ. Expression of membrane-associated human chorionic gonadotropin, its subunits, and fragments by cultured human cancer cells. *Cancer.* 1992;69:1829–1842.

(65)  Roberts W. *Collected Contributions on Digestion and Diet.* 2nd ed. London: Smith, Elder & Co.; 1897.

(66)  Gurchot C. The trophoblast theory of cancer (John Beard, 1857–1924) revisited. *Oncology.* 1975;31:310–333.

(67)  Beard J. The scientific criterion of a malignant tumor. *Med Rec.* 1907;71:24–25.

(68)  Beard J. The action of trypsin upon the living cells of Jensen's mouse-tumour. *Br Med J.* 1906;1:140–141.

(69)  Rice CC. Treatment of cancer of the larynx by subcutaneous injection of pancreatic extract (trypsin). *Med Rec.* 1906;70:812–816.

(70)  Campbell JT. Trypsin treatment of a case of malignant disease. *J Am Med Assoc.* 1907;48:225–226.

(71)  Cutfield A. Trypsin treatment in malignant disease. *Br Med J.* 1907;2:525.

(72)  Cleaves MA. Pancreatic ferments in the treatment of cancer and their role in prophylaxis. *Med Rec.* 1906;70:918.

(73)  Golley FB. Two cases of cancer treated by the injection of pancreatic extract. *Med Rec.* 1906;70:918–919.

(74)  Weinstein JW. Dr. Beard's theory in the crucible of test. An experimental study of the trypsin treatment in cancer. *N Y State J Med.* 1908;9:400–402.

(75) Saleeby CW. Cancer—can it be cured? *McClure's Magazine*. 1906; 27:438–445.

(76) Saleeby CW. *The Conquest of Cancer*. New York, NY: Frederick A. Stokes Company; 1907.

(77) Conquest of cancer. *New York Times* January 4, 1908.

(78) Beard J. The system of branchial sense-organs and their associated ganglia in ichthyopsida. *Quart J Micr Sci*. 1885.

(79) Zwaka TP, Thomson JA. A germ cell origin of embryonic stem cells? *Development*. 2005;132:227–233.

(80) Colombo C, Maiavacca R, Ronchi M et al. Serum levels of immunoreactive trypsin during development: comparison with levels of lipase and amylase. *J Pediatr Gastroenterol Nutr*. 1989;9:194–199.

(81) Terada T, Nakanuma Y. Expression of pancreatic enzymes (alpha-amylase, trypsinogen, and lipase) during human liver development and maturation. *Gastroenterology*. 1995;108:1236–1245.

(82) Koop H. Serum levels of pancreatic enzymes and their clinical significance. *Clin Gastroenterol*. 1984;13:739–761.

(83) Guyton AC, Hall JE. *Textbook of Medical Physiology*. 10th ed. Philadelphia, PA: W.B. Saunders Company; 2000.

(84) Porter W. Some practical suggestions on the treatment of diphtheria. *J Am Med Assoc*. 1886;7:454–455.

(85) *Fairchild's Hand-Book of the Digestive Ferments*. New York, NY: Fairchild Bros. & Foster; 1898.

(86) Beard J. Trypsin and amylopsin in cancer. *Med Rec*. 1906;69:1020.

(87) Levin E. Production of dried, defatted enzymatic material. *U S Patent Office*. 1950;1–7.

(88) Hald PT. Comparative researches on the tryptic strength of different trypsin preparations and on their action on the human body. *Lancet*. 1907;170:1371–1375.

(89) Wilhelm Conrad Röntgen—biography. http://nobelprize.org/nobel_prizes/physics/laureates/1901/rontgen-bio.html. Accessed June 26, 2008.

(90) Wilhelm Conrad Röntgen. http://en.wikipedia.org/wiki/Wilhelm_Rontgen. Accessed June 26, 2008.

(91) Marie Curie. http://en.wikipedia.org/wiki/Marie_Curie. Accessed June 26, 2008.

(92) Morse FL. Treatment of cancer with pancreatic extract. *Wkly Bull St Louis Med Soc*. 1934;28:599–603.

(93) Shively FL. *Multiple Proteolytic Enzyme Therapy of Cancer*. Dayton, OH: John-Watson Printing and Bookbinding Co.; 1969.

(94) Kelley WD. *One Answer to Cancer*. Los Angeles, CA: Cancer Book House; 1969.

(95) Howell EH. *Food Enzymes for Health & Longevity*. Woodstock Valley, CT: Omangod Press; 1980.

(96) Regan PT, Malagelada JR, DiMagno EP, Glanzman SL, Go VL. Comparative effects of antacids, cimetidine and enteric coating on the therapeutic response to oral enzymes in severe pancreatic insufficiency. *N Engl J Med*. 1977;297:854–858.

(97)   Graham DY. An enteric-coated pancreatic enzyme preparation that works. *Dig Dis Sci.* 1979;24:906–909.

(98)   Dutta SK, Rubin J, Harvey J. Comparative evaluation of the therapeutic efficacy of a pH- sensitive enteric coated pancreatic enzyme preparation with conventional pancreatic enzyme therapy in the treatment of exocrine pancreatic insufficiency. *Gastroenterology.* 1983;84:476–482.

(99)   Andren-Sandberg A. Theory and practice in the individualization of oral pancreatic enzyme administration for chronic pancreatitis. *Int J Pancreatol.* 1989;5 Suppl:51–62.

(100)  Moskvichyov BV, Komarov EV, Ivanova GP. Study of trypsin thermodenaturation process. *Enzyme Microb Tech.* 1986;8:498–502.

(101)  Legg EF, Spencer AM. Studies on the stability of pancreatic enzymes in duodenal fluid to storage temperature and pH. *Clin Chim Acta.* 1975;65:175–179.

(102)  Rothman S, Liebow C, Isenman L. Conservation of digestive enzymes. *Physiol Rev.* 2002;82:1–18.

(103)  Liebow C, Rothman SS. Enteropancreatic circulation of digestive enzymes. *Science.* 1975;189:472–474.

(104)  Thomson M, Clague A, Cleghorn GJ, Shepherd RW. Comparative in vitro and in vivo studies of enteric-coated pancrelipase preparations for pancreatic insufficiency. *J Pediatr Gastroenterol Nutr.* 1993;17:407–413.

(105)  Questions and answers on exocrine pancreatic insufficiency drug products. http://www.fda.gov/CDER/DRUG/infopage/pancreatic_drugs/pancreatic_QA.htm. Accessed June 25, 2008.

(106)  FitzSimmons SC, Burkhart GA, Borowitz D et al. High-dose pancreatic-enzyme supplements and fibrosing colonopathy in children with cystic fibrosis. *N Engl J Med.* 1997;336:1283–1289.

(107)  FDA requires pancreatic extract manufacturers to submit marketing applications. http://www.fda.gov/bbs/topics/news/2004/NEW01058.html. Accessed June 25, 2008.

(108)  Muller DP, Ghale GK. Stability of pancreatic enzyme activities in duodenal juice after pancreatic stimulation by a test meal or exogenous hormones. *Ann Clin Biochem.* 1982;19: 89–93.

(109)  Novak JF, Trnka F. Proenzyme therapy of cancer. *Anticancer Res.* 2005;25:1157–1177.

(110)  Trujillo ME, Scherer PE. Adipose tissue-derived factors: impact on health and disease. *Endocr Rev.* 2006;27:762–778.

(111)  Gonzalez NJ. *One Man Alone; An Investigation of Nutrition, Cancer, and William Donald Kelley.* New York, NY: New Spring Press; 2010.

(112)  DeVita VT, Jr., Hellman S, Rosenberg SA, editors. *Cancer: Principles & Practice of Oncology.* 1st ed. Philadelphia, PA: J.B. Lippincott Company; 1982.

(113)  Petersdorf RG, Adams RD, Braunwald E, Isselbacher KJ, Martin JB, Wilson JD, editors. *Harrison's Principles of Internal Medicine.* 10th ed. New York, NY: McGraw-Hill Book Company; 1983.

(114)  Harvey AM, Johns RJ, McKusick VA, Owens AH, Ross RS, editors. *The Principles and Practice of Medicine.* 20th ed. New York, NY: Appleton-Century-Crofts; 1980.

(115)  Gonzalez NJ, Isaacs LL. Evaluation of pancreatic proteolytic enzyme treatment of adenocarcinoma of the pancreas, with nutrition and detoxification support. *Nutr Cancer.* 1999;33:117–124.

(116) Burris HA, Moore MJ, Andersen J et al. Improvements in survival and clinical benefit with gemcitabine as first-line therapy for patients with advanced pancreas cancer: a randomized trial. *J Clin Oncol.* 1997;15:2403–2413.

(117) Saruc M, Standop S, Standop J et al. Pancreatic enzyme extract improves survival in murine pancreatic cancer. *Pancreas.* 2004;28:401–412.

(118) Liener IE, Goodale RL, Deshmukh A et al. Effect of a trypsin inhibitor from soybeans (Bowman-Birk) on the secretory activity of the human pancreas. *Gastroenterology.* 1988;94:419–427.

(119) Lentzsch S, Reichardt P, Weber F, Budach V, Dorken B. Brain metastases in breast cancer: prognostic factors and management. *Eur J Cancer.* 1999;35:580–585.

(120) Eichbaum MH, Kaltwasser M, Bruckner T, de Rossi TM, Schneeweiss A, Sohn C. Prognostic factors for patients with liver metastases from breast cancer. *Breast Cancer Res Treat.* 2006;96:53–62.

# Index

Illustrations are indicated by *italic page references*

# About the Authors

**Nicholas J. Gonzalez, M.D.:** Dr. Gonzalez graduated from Brown University, Phi Beta Kappa, magna cum laude with a degree in English Literature. He worked as a journalist, first at Time Inc., before pursuing premedical studies at Columbia University. He received his medical degree from Cornell University Medical College in 1983. During a postgraduate immunology fellowship under Dr. Robert A. Good, considered the father of modern immunology, Dr. Gonzalez investigated the nutritional cancer treatment developed by the dentist Dr. William Kelley. Dr. Gonzalez's research has been funded by The Procter & Gamble Company, Nestlé, and the National Cancer Institute/National Institutes of Health. Since 1987, Dr. Gonzalez has been in private practice in New York City treating cancer and other degenerative diseases with an enzyme-based nutritional regimen. He is in the process of publishing a series of books, of which *Trophoblast* is the first. For more information on his practice or his books, see his website at www.dr-gonzalez.com.

**Linda L. Isaacs, M.D.:** Dr. Isaacs graduated from the University of Kentucky, Phi Beta Kappa with High Distinction, and subsequently received her medical degree from Vanderbilt University School of Medicine. She completed a residency in Internal Medicine at the Department of Veteran's Affairs Medical Center at New York University Medical School and is Board Certified in Internal Medicine. Since 1985, Dr. Isaacs has been working with Dr. Gonzalez in his private practice and research efforts.

To learn more about Dr. Nicholas Gonzalez's research and medical practice, please visit:

www.dr-gonzalez.com
or call 212–213–3337

Dr. Gonzalez treats many types of cancer and other illnesses such as allergies, autoimmune disorders and chronic fatigue.

For other published works and recordings by Dr. Gonzalez, please contact New Spring Press.

Thank you for your interest!

---

NEW SPRING PRESS
PO Box 200
New York, NY 10156

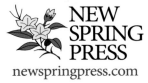

NEW
SPRING
PRESS
newspringpress.com